50/9

WITHDRAWN

D1556776

LIVERPOOL POLYTECHNIC LIBRARY

3 1111 00433 5590

Impacts on Nutrition and Health

World Review of Nutrition and Dietetics

Vol. 65

Series Editor
Artemis P. Simopoulos, Washington, D.C.

Advisory Board

Åke Bruce, Sweden
Ji Di Chen, China
Jean-Claude Dillon, France
J.E. Dutra de Oliveira, Brazil
Claudio Galli, Italy
G. Gopalan, India
Demetre Labadarios, South Africa
Eleazar Lara-Pantin, Venezuela
Paul J. Nestel, Australia
Jana Pařizková, Czechoslovakia
Konstantin Pavlou, Greece
A. Rérat, France
George Rhoads, United States
V. Rogozkin, USSR
F.J. Stare, United States
Naomi Trostler, Israel

Members Emeriti, Advisory Board

J. Ganguly, India
C. den Hartog, Netherlands
D.M. Hegsted, United States

KARGER

Basel · München · Paris · London · NewYork · New Delhi · Bangkok · Singapore · Tokyo · Sydney

Impacts on Nutrition and Health

Volume Editor
Artemis P. Simopoulos
The Center for Genetics, Nutrition and Health, American Association for
World Health, Washington, D.C.

31 figures and 23 tables, 1991

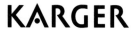

Basel · München · Paris · London · NewYork · New Delhi · Bangkok · Singapore · Tokyo · Sydney

World Review of Nutrition and Dietetics

Library of Congress Cataloging-in-Publication Data
Impacts on nutrition and health / volume editor, Artemis P. Simopoulos.
(World review of nutrition and dietetics; vol. 65)
Includes bibliographical references.
Includes index.
1. Nutrition. 2. Nutritionally induced diseases. 3. Health.
I. Simopoulos, Artemis P., 1933– . II. Series.
[DNLM: 1. Health. 2. Nutrition.]
ISBN 3–8055–5266–1

Bibliographic Indices
This publication is listed in bibliographic services, including Current Contents® and Index Medicus.

Drug Dosage
The authors and the publisher have exerted every effort to ensure that drug selection and dosage set forth in this text are in accord with current recommendations and practice at the time of publication. However, in view of ongoing research, changes in government regulations, and the constant flow of information relating to drug therapy and drug reactions, the reader is urged to check the package insert for each drug for any change in indications and dosage and for added warnings and precautions. This is particularly important when the recommended agent is a new and/or infrequently employed drug.

All rights reserved.
No part of this publication may be translated into other languages, reproduced or utilized in any form or by any means, electronic or mechanical, including photocopying, recording, microcopying, or by any information storage and retrieval system, without permission in writing from the publisher.

© Copyright 1991 by S. Karger AG, P.O. Box, CH–4009 Basel (Switzerland)
Printed in Switzerland by Thür AG Offsetdruck, Pratteln
ISBN 3–8055–5266–1

Contents

Contents

Simopoulos AP (ed): Impacts on Nutrition and Health.
World Rev Nutr Diet. Basel, Karger, 1991, vol 65, pp 1–37

Sorbitol and Dental Caries

Dowen Birkhed[a], *Albert Bär*[b]

[a] Department of Cariology, University of Göteborg, Sweden, and
[b] Bioresco Ltd., Binningen, Switzerland

Contents

Sugar, Sugar Substitutes and Dental Caries

On the basis of numerous clinical and nonclinical studies it is by now well established that dietary sugars play a crucial role in the development of dental caries [1–4]. A direct, quantitative relationship between sugar consumption and caries cannot be established because of positively or negatively interfering effects of various other host- and environment-related factors, but a trend analysis of sugar consumption and caries incidence supports the view that the presently consumed levels of sugars contribute significantly to caries in most industrialized, and in many developing countries [1, 5–8]. On the other hand, recent reports on a decline in caries have amply documented the efficacy of preventive measures – particularly the application of fluorides – on dental health, and have thereby somewhat alleviated previous concerns about the potential adverse dental effects of sugars [9]. However, one would be misled to conclude from a reported 30–80% reduction of caries in children of some countries that this disease is generally no longer a serious health problem. In fact, there is good evidence that occlusal and proximal tooth surfaces profited less from the decline in caries [10, 11]. It also appears that a substantial subset of children continues to exhibit a high incidence of tooth decay [12–14]. Moreover, nearly all epidemiological studies on caries have concentrated on schoolchildren, and comparatively little is, therefore, known about present trends in oral health of the older population. In this regard, a few recent studies suggest that the caries incidence in adults is still considerable [14–16] and that in the future, root caries may occur more frequently in the older population because more teeth are retained for longer periods of time [17]. Therefore, dietary counselling remains to be an important element of caries prevention in addition to instruction in oral hygiene and continued fluoride application.

Traditionally, advice to change eating patterns has concentrated on the reduction of readily fermentable foods eaten between meals, particularly of sugary foods. Although such measures have been urged by dentists during decades, their practical value remained limited. Recent investigations on dietary habits and snacking suggest that the consumption of sweets is in fact still increasing [18]. In principle, the consumers are increasingly aware about the association of good nutrition and good health, and they are prepared to change long-established eating habits if particular foods or food ingredients are perceived to be unhealthy. However, many examples demonstrate that the consumer is willing to change his dietary habits and to refrain from certain products only if acceptable alternatives are available on the market. For this reason, it appears logical to put even more emphasis on replacing sugars with noncariogenic alternative sweeteners, especially in those foods and drinks that are consumed frequently and that are known to have a high cariogenic potential.

Among the bulk sugar substitutes that are currently used in confectionery, chewing gum, chocolate, jam, jellies and other sweets, sorbitol plays an eminent role because of its good technological properties (sweetness, hygroscopicity, solubility), its well-established safety and regulatory acceptance, and its comparatively low price. Reliable data on the present consumption of sugar-free confectionery and of sorbitol are scarce. However, it is known that in 1988 sugar-free products reached a marked share of 15.1% of the total confectionery market in Switzerland where consumers are particularly aware of the advantages of such products because of a coordinated promotional effort from industry and the dental institutes. From these data, a daily intake of about 0.5 g sorbitol/day/person may be estimated. This value corresponds quite well with the result of a Finnish study in which a daily intake of 0.4 g/day was calculated [19]. At a first glance, these values appear to be too low to be of any relevance in terms of sugar substitution and caries prevention. However, it shoud be noted that only a certain percentage of the total population consumes sweet snacks regularly, and that the daily intake may be considerably higher for such regular and heavy users of sweets, which profit most from reducing the frequency and amount of sugar exposure by favouring sugar-free brands over the more traditional, cariogenic sweets.

In view of the health advantages which the consumer expects to obtain from sugar-free sweets, in consideration of the widespread use of sorbitol in such products, and in recognition of a few recent, somewhat critical opinions on this sugar substitute, it seems appropriate to review the caries-related aspects of sorbitol on basis of the available scientific data.

Metabolism and Safety Profile of Sorbitol

Sorbitol has been found in various fruits and vegetables as well as – in trace amounts – in the human organism [20–23]. Ingested sorbitol is absorbed slowly and incompletely from the gut by passive diffusion. The fraction which is absorbed, reaches the liver with the portal vein blood where it is readily metabolized. In an initial dehydrogenation step, sorbitol is converted by sorbitol dehydrogenase to fructose which, after phosphorylation by fructokinase to fructose-1-phosphate, is channeled into the glycolytic pathway. Since the hepatic metabolism proceeds at a rate which exceeds the intestinal diffusion rate by far, the blood and tissue levels of sorbitol are negligibly low. Experiments with normal and diabetic rats have shown that the dietary administration of sorbitol has no effect on the sorbitol levels of the eye lens and the kidney [24, 25].

The fraction of sorbitol which escapes absorption in the small intestine reaches the microbially colonized distal parts of the gut where rapid fermentation takes place. The breakdown products of this bacterial metabolism are mainly acetic, propionic and butyric acid, lactic acid, carbon dioxide and small amounts of methane [26]. The volatile fatty acids formed are efficiently absorbed in the colon and are then utilized for gluconeogenesis (propionic acid) and for lipid formation (acetic and butyric acid).

On basis of a large number of toxicological, biochemical and clinical investigations, the safety of sorbitol has been assessed by different national and international regulatory authorities. On an international level, the Joint FAO/WHO Expert Committee on Food Additives (JECFA) has allocated an Acceptable Daily Intake (ADI) 'not specified' for sorbitol in 1982 [27]. Similarly, the Scientific Committee for Food for the European Economic Community (SCF-EEC) proposed 'acceptance' of this polyol in 1984. On a national level, sorbitol is approved for foods, cosmetics, and pharmaceuticals in over 40 countries. In the US, the Code of Federal Regulations (21 CFR 184.1835) lists sorbitol as a Generally Recognized as Safe (GRAS) substance and gives guidelines for the use of sorbitol as a food ingredient.

The Life Sciences Research Office (LSRO) Select Committee on GRAS Substances evaluated the health aspects of sorbitol as part of a comprehensive review by the US Food and Drug Administration (FDA) on the safety of GRAS food ingredients in 1972, and an additional LSRO report on sorbitol was prepared in 1979 [28]. The most recent review of certain toxicological data was conducted in 1986 by the Federation of the American Scientists for Experimental Biology (FASEB) at the request of the FDA [29]. The published conclusions of this Expert group indicates that the use of sorbitol is not expected to present any significant risk to human health. The report also supports the view that sorbitol has a similar safety profile as other sugar alcohols and lactose which are widely used in our daily food supply.

The tolerance of humans to high oral doses of sorbitol has been investigated in numerous studies with healthy and diabetic volunteers. Adverse changes of clinical parameters were generally not observed. However, transient laxation and gastrointestinal discomfort may be experienced after the consumption of high doses of sorbitol. Such side effects are generally observed after intake of sugar alcohols and slowly digestible carbohydrates (e.g., lactose, fruit juices). Persons with an individual, particular sensitivity to such effects may respond to even relatively low doses of these products (5–10 g). However, because of an almost immediate onset of the symptoms, these sensitive subjects are normally aware of their condition and avoid therefore corresponding foods. It is considered that the slow absorption of sorbitol and similar compounds from the gut results in an osmotic imbalance which may be the cause of intestinal disturbance. From a practical point of view, it is important that these effects are readily reversible upon reduction of the amounts of sugar alcohol consumed [30, 31]. Tolerance usually develops with continued exposure. In recognition of these facts, the FDA has determined that food providing daily ingestion of 50 g or more of sorbitol must bear the label statement 'Excess consumption may have a laxative effect'. However, the agency also pointed out that it is unlikely that diarrhoea will occur in persons who consume sorbitol-containing food under ordinary circumstances.

Assessment of the Cariogenic Potential of Sorbitol

Models for Assessing Cariogenic Potential
Model systems to assess the cariogenic potential of foods and food ingredients in short-term experiments include essentially three main methods. The first approach, originated by Stephan [32] in 1940, involves the measurement of pH in dental plaque. Meanwhile, different test systems have been developed from the original system but the method which has gained most favour is the telemetric measurement of plaque pH with an indwelling electrode [33]. A second approach relies on the formation of dental caries in experimental animals, mainly in rats and hamsters and, more rarely, in monkeys. While plaque pH measurement provides only information on the acidogenicity of a test food or a test substance, the animal experiment allows to investigate the relative importance of other factors as well, such as the frequency of exposure, the dose, and the presence of other food components [34]. Finally, a third category of assessment methods is based upon enamel de- and remineralization phenomena which may be examined under in vitro or in vivo conditions [35].

Although all three methods provide some information about the cariogenic potential of a test substance, the true cariogenicity of a given food can by definition be determined in long-term caries studies in man only. Due to the high cost and the various difficulties associated with the design, experimental conduct and statistical analysis of such trials, respective data are, however, very scarce. Therefore, assessment of the cariogenic potential has normally to rely on the results of short-term experiments whereby the limitations of the applied models must be appropriately taken into account if extrapolations to the cariogenicity in humans are to be made.

Fermentability of Sorbitol by Oral Microorganisms

In vitro Fermentation of Sorbitol by Pure Strains of Oral Microorganisms. Most of the microorganisms that dominate in human plaque and in saliva cannot utilize sorbitol as a source of carbon and energy [36–39]. However, a majority of the strains of *Streptococcus mutans,* lactobacilli, and some less frequently encountered oral microorganisms, such as propionibacteria and enterococci, do ferment sorbitol [36, 37, 40–50]. A few strains of Actinomyces, *Streptococcus sanguis* and *Streptococcus mitior* also have this ability [42, 51, 52].

Mutans streptococci play a particularly prominent role in the formation of dental caries. Consequently, most studies on the fermentation of sorbitol by oral microorganisms have been conducted with isolated strains of this species. Studies with intact cells and with cell extracts of *S. mutans* indicate that the uptake and phosphorylation of sorbitol are mediated by a phosphotransferase system. The delivered intracellular sorbitol-6-P is subsequently oxidized to fructose-6-P by a sorbitol-6-P dehydrogenase [53–55]. Fructose-6-P is further degraded through the Emden-Meyerhof pathway. Finally, pyruvate is converted to lactate, formate, acetate and ethanol [56–58]. In a couple of investigations it has been demonstrated that *S. sanguis, S. mitior* and *S. mutans* metabolize sorbitol to a different spectrum of end products under anaerobic and aerobic conditions [57–60]. Pyruvate formate lyase (PFL), which catalyzes the first step of the conversion of pyruvate to volatile compounds (formate, acetate, ethanol), is an extremely oxygen-sensitive enzyme. Consequently, anaerobically grown *S. mutans* ferment sorbitol mainly into formate and ethanol with traces of lactate and acetate also occurring. After exposure to oxygen, however, the same cells ferment sorbitol at a much slower rate whereby only lactate is formed in detectable amounts [57, 58, 60]. A corresponding but less pronounced effect was observed for *S. sanguis* which seems to possess some mechanism to protect its PFL from oxidative inactivation [57, 58].

While concern has been expressed that the observed fermentability of sorbitol, particularly by *S. mutans,* may limit the value of sorbitol as a noncariogenic sugar substitute, it is essential to bear in mind that there are fundamental differences between the fermentation of sucrose and sorbitol by *S. mutans* and other sorbitol-fermenting microorganisms.

First of all, it is well established that the fermentation of sorbitol proceeds at a rather slow rate [39, 55, 56], and that the final pH in liquid cultures normally does not reach such low levels as are regularly seen with glucose or sucrose [39, 48, 49, 52, 61–64]. Since the oral microflora is usually exposed to sorbitol in vivo for short periods of time only, and since sorbitol unlike carbohydrates cannot be converted to polysaccharides serving as substrate storage compounds, it appears unlikely that the fermentation of sorbitol yields acids in relevant amounts. The results of in vivo plaque pH measurements support this view as will be outlined in the following section of this paper in more detail.

Second, it has been found that both the sorbitol-specific phosphotransferase and the sorbitol dehydrogenase represent inducible enzymes which are synthesized only when the bacteria are exposed to sorbitol for a sufficient period of time [52, 65, 66]. This also means that in the presence of glucose, the bacterial metabolism is rapidly switched back to the metabolic utilization of this more easily available energy source. At the same time the sorbitol transport and catabolism is repressed [53, 55]. Because of (1) the constant presence of low levels of glucose in saliva, (2) the intermittent release of larger amounts of glucose from alimentary starch by salivary amylase, and (3) the mobilization of glucose from polysaccharide reserves, it is questionable whether a significant sorbitol-catabolic activity may be maintained by plaque and salivary bacteria over relevant periods of time.

Third, it must be noticed that the degradation of sorbitol yields a quantitatively different profile of fermentation end products than the catabolism of glucose and sucrose (fig. 1). Under anaerobic conditions, lactic acid is the major product of glucose fermentation while formate and acetate are formed in relatively small amounts. Sorbitol, on the other hand, yields considerable amounts of ethanol and formate but only a smaller proportion of lactic acid [56, 58, 66a, b]. This observation is relevant because lactic acid exerts a stronger demineralizing effect on tooth enamel than the other volatile fermentation end products.

Fourth, there is no evidence that sorbitol may be used for the production of insoluble extracellular polysaccharides which play an important role in the formation and adhesion of dental plaque [38, 39, 67]. On the other hand, there is also no evidence that sorbitol inhibits polysaccharide formation as it has been shown for fructose and certain other carbohy-

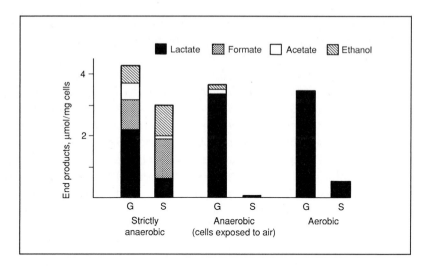

Fig. 1. Fermentation end products of sorbitol-grown cells of *S. mutans* with sorbitol (S) or glucose (G) [adapted from 95].

drates [68]. A slight enhancing effect of sorbitol on the sucrose-derived formation of soluble and insoluble polysaccharides by *S. mutans* in vitro has probably no clinical relevance [69].

In conclusion, it does not appear justified to question the use of sorbitol as a sugar substitute on the mere basis that certain oral microorganisms, including *S. mutans,* are able to produce some acid from sorbitol in vitro.

In vitro Fermentation of Sorbitol by a Mixed Oral Flora. For the investigation of metabolic pathways and regulation mechanisms, experiments with isolated bacterial strains provide valuable information. For an assessment of the cariogenic potential of different substrates, however, studies with a mixed oral flora yield more relevant results.

Numerous experiments have been carried out in which dental plaque or salivary microorganisms were incubated in the presence of sorbitol. In a very early study with saliva, it was shown that acid was produced from sorbitol at a much lower rate than from glucose or sucrose under aerobic or anaerobic conditions. The author also noted that even after incubation for 24 h, the pH of the mixture did not reach critical levels for enamel decal-

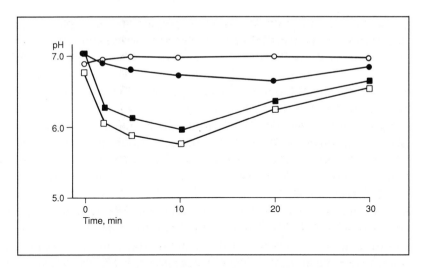

Fig. 2. Plaque pH after a 30 s mouth rinse with 10% solutions of glucose (□) and sorbitol (○) before and with glucose (■) and sorbitol (●) after a 6-week period with frequent daily mouth rinses with sorbitol (means of 18 subjects) [from 74].

cification [40]. Subsequent experiments with saliva or with plaque suspensions of higher bacterial density gave similar results [60, 62, 69, 70–79]. In general, it was found that the fermentation rate of sorbitol amounted to about 15–25% of that of glucose or sucrose [72, 76, 79]. However, considerably lower [78] and higher [60] values have also been reported.

As in the above mentioned experiments with pure cultures [39, 49, 61, 62], it was consistently found that the metabolically active phase was preceded by a more or less pronounced lag period. It was also confirmed that lactic acid was only a minor end product of sorbitol fermentation [60, 69, 79].

In vivo Fermentation of Sorbitol by Plaque in situ. Changes of plaque pH in vivo after rinses with solutions of sorbitol or after consumption of sorbitol-based sweets have been studied by different groups (fig. 2) [74, 80–86]. The conclusion of all these experiments is that plaque pH drops only marginally, if at all, and that in no one instance, a critically low plaque pH was obtained as a result of sorbitol fermentation. Occasionally, even an increase of plaque pH was observed probably due to stimulated salivation [81, 82, 85]. This effect was particularly pronounced if chewing gum was used as a vehicle for sorbitol [87].

In line with these results, comparative quantitation of plaque organic acids formed in vivo in the course of chewing sucrose and sorbitol-mannitol-containing gums revealed that the hexitol gum did not generate any additional lactic, formic, butyric, propionic, acetic or pyruvic acid beyond baseline (0 time) values. In contrast, sucrose-containing gum produced significant increases in lactic and butyric acids [88]. Using a different approach, the fermentability of sorbitol by the total oral microflora (in plaque and saliva, on tongue and mucosa) was estimated by measuring microbially formed hydrogen in the exhaled air before and after a rinse with solutions of sorbitol and other sweeteners. The results demonstrate that H_2 expiration increased to 10 times the fasting levels after a sucrose or glucose challenge, while after sorbitol and mannitol an increase of 50% only was noted [89]. This novel method represents an interesting tool for assessing the fermentability of different substrates in vivo because it is noninvasive and because the H_2 exchange proceeds at a fast rate even from deeper layers of the plaque. On the other hand, the results do not provide direct, quantitative information about the formation of acid which is more relevant for caries prediction.

At present, plaque pH telemetry represents probably the best-suited method for the assessment of acid formation by plaque in situ [33, 90]. Using this technique, the acidogenicity of pure sorbitol solutions and of sorbitol-sweeetened foods has been examined in countless tests. Already the first experiments that were undertaken with this method included tests on sorbitol [91, 92]. These and all subsequent corresponding investigations demonstrate consistently that the consumption of sorbitol is not associated with an acidification of dental plaque that would be indicative of a cariogenic risk [33, 93].

Concluding Remarks on Fermentation Tests. On basis of various fermentation tests, different authors have arrived at different conclusions about the cariogenic potential of sorbitol. Although there seems to be consensus that sorbitol is much less cariogenic than sucrose, some investigators have argued that the observed acidogenicity makes the use of sorbitol for the production of dentally safe sweets questionable [70, 94]. It has even been suggested that in the mentioned experiments the acidogenicity of sorbitol may have been underestimated because the oral bacteria were exposed to air (oxygen) during preparation [95]. However, in consideration of the same results, others have taken a more neutral position [79], or they have even concluded that sorbitol does not bear any significant cariogenic risk because of the different reasons mentioned above [55].

In our opinion, in vitro studies with mixed oral flora may well provide some estimates about the relative acidogenicity of different carbohydrates and sugar alcohols. However, for predicting relative cariogenicity the model is inappropriate for the following reasons. First the microorganisms are exposed in vitro to the test compounds for long periods of time while under the more relevant in vivo conditions only relatively short pulses – alternated with exposure to other nutrients – are available to the bacteria. Second, all natural defense and repair mechanisms that may play an important role in vivo are completely eliminated from the mentioned laboratory test systems. For these reasons, the in vitro acidogenicity tests may rather overestimate than underestimate the true cariogenic potential of a test compound. More reliable data may be obtained only from in vivo studies with plaque in situ which take these factors into account at least to some extent.

Are There Adaptive Changes in Dental Plaque upon Prolonged Exposure to Sorbitol?

Mechanisms of Adaptation

It is a well-known phenomenon in microbiology that microorganisms can alter their phenotype and can become capable of fermenting new and less readily accessible substrates if the traditional sources of energy and carbon atoms are exhausted or if they are available in limited amounts only.

A well-documented example for the induction of a sorbitol-degrading enzyme system is presented by the intestinal microflora which, upon continued exposure to sorbitol for a few days, acquires the ability to effectively ferment this normally not present substrate. Considering the biological significance and hence the widespread occurrence of such inductive changes, it has been discussed whether the oral microflora may adapt to the presence of sorbitol in a similar way [94, 96, 97]. If this was the case, the advantages of sorbitol as a hypoacidogenic sugar substitute would get lost at least partly because an enhanced acid formation would result.

Theoretically, an adaptation of the oral microflora to sorbitol can occur not only as a result of an enzyme induction but also by a raise in the number of microorganisms which possess constitutive enzymes for sorbitol degradation and which consequently have an ecological advantage if sorbitol is offered frequently as an energy source. In addition, other members of the oral cavity could gain the ability to ferment sorbitol by genetic transfer of genomes from sorbitol-fermenting bacteria. Experiments in vitro indeed suggest that markers for sorbitol metabolism can be transferred between oral bacteria, but since this transfer seems to be limited to certain pairs of donor/recipient strains, this observation has probably little practical relevance [65]. Similarly, the possibility of sequential mutational events appears rather remote.

Metabolic Changes in Dental Plaque

The effects of sorbitol on plaque accumulation as well as the possibility of sorbitol-induced metabolic and ecological changes of the plaque flora have been examined in different in vivo studies with human volunteers [98–112] and in one experiment with monkeys [113]. More recent studies have been conducted in particular risk groups, such as in persons with low salivary secretion rate [114], children with fixed orthodontic appliances [86], and diabetic patients [115]. Some case reports on the plaque characteristics of heavy sorbitol consumers have been published as well [116, 117, 121].

Studies on the potential microbial adaptation to sorbitol have mainly focused on the acid formation from sorbitol by dental plaque before and after a period with frequent sorbitol consumption whereby sorbitol was usually administered with chewing gum, rinsing solutions, candies, or toothpaste. The results of all these studies are consistent to the extent that even after long-term exposure to sorbitol the acid formation from sorbitol does not result in plaque pH levels and acid formation rates which were indicative of a cariogenic risk. However, with regard to the more subtle effects, less agreement is observed.

In a study with a 4 times daily consumption of Lycasin®, maltitol-, sorbitol-, or xylitol-based lozenges for 3 months, there were no significant differences between the plaque pH changes induced by rinsing with solutions of the respective sugar alcohols [99]. Similar results were obtained in a study on patients with fixed orthodontic appliances in which no significant change in plaque pH was noted in response to the consumption of a sorbitol gum either before or after a 12-week period of regular gum consumption (3 sticks/day) [86]. Similarly, in a study on monkeys which received daily amounts of 30 g sorbitol with their diet for 2 years, no increased fall in plaque pH was noted [113]. On the other hand, a slight indication for an adaptation of the plaque to sorbitol as a fermentable substrate is provided by a study in which healthy volunteers consumed xylitol-, xylitol/sorbitol-, or sorbitol-sweetened chewing gums for periods of 4 days each. It was found that exposure to sorbitol resulted in slightly but significantly lower plaque pH values after the period with sorbitol consumption than after the period with xylitol consumption (10 times 2 sticks of chewing gum/day) [108].

More clear-cut indications of a sorbitol-related adaptation stem from a study on persons with low salivary secretion rate. After a 4-week period with regular sorbitol rinsing (10–15 times/day), the acid production from sorbitol increased in vivo and in vitro [114a]. Since individuals with dry mouth have a reduced ability to neutralize plaque acids [118] and since they therefore harbour a large number of aciduric organisms in dental plaque [119], it might be hypothesized that the adaptation procedure boosted mainly the sorbitol-utilizing enzyme system of S. mutans and lactobacilli which are already highly prevalent in xerostomic patients.

Taken together, these results indicate that even a frequent use of sorbitol does not cause biochemical changes in dental plaque which can predispose to caries development except perhaps in dry mouth patients with extremely frequent exposure to sorbitol. In all other cases, the slight increase in acid production from sorbitol that may occur, does not reach critical levels probably because the normal exposure to more readily available substrates efficiently represses the induction of a sorbitol-degrading enzyme system.

Ecological Shifts in Dental Plaque

Several investigators have tried to determine whether frequent sorbitol exposure may select for sorbitol-fermenting microorganisms such as S. mutans and/or lactobacilli in plaque. In one study involving monkeys [113], the animals were fed diets containing sorbitol or sucrose for alternating 3- to 4-week periods. Determination of the plaque S. mutans levels revealed that an explosive increase in S. mutans occurred when the animals were switched from a sorbitol-containing diet to a diet providing about 35 g/day sucrose. When the animals were subsequently returned to the sucrose-free but sorbitol-supplemented diet, the numbers of S. mutans in plaque decreased within 3 weeks to almost zero. This study suggested that the prominence of S. mutans in the plaque was exclusively sucrose-dependent and that high population density in plaque could not be sustained by sorbitol.

In humans, the effect of sorbitol (and xylitol) on plaque and saliva levels of *S. mutans* was also tested. In one study, the consumption of lozenges with 0.5 g sorbitol, taken 4 times/day, was not associated with changes in the proportions of *S. mutans* and lactobacilli in the volunteers' plaque [99]. In another study, high salivary levels of lactobaccili were found more frequently in children who consumed sorbitol-sweetened chocolates for 2 years than in children who consumed ordinary chocolate with sucrose [120]. However, different results have also been reported. For example, it was observed that persons who had consumed on average 6.7 sorbitol-containing foods/day for at least 2 years, had slightly increased numbers of *S. mutans* in saliva, compared to a nonselected control group. Sorbitol-fermenting varieties of *S. sanguis*, *S. mitior* and *S. salivarius* were also found in the saliva samples of the sorbitol consumers [121]. These observations parallel those of other investigators who also detected high numbers of *S. mutans* in subjects with frequent sorbitol consumption [104, 116, 117].

For the time being, there are only few experimental studies which suggest that a frequent consumption of sorbitol may increase the plaque and saliva levels of *S. mutans* under certain conditions. In a first study, healthy volunteers were kept on a carbohydrate-free diet while they ate xylitol- or sorbitol-sweetened candies for 4 days at a frequency of 6 candies/day. A significant increase in the porportion of anaerobic sorbitol-fermenting bacteria was detected in the sorbitol test group but the authors stressed the fact that only a small proportion of the plaque bacteria was able to ferment sorbitol [106]. Since the volunteers were kept on a carbohydrate-free diet, the adaptive pressure for developing a sorbitol-degrading enzyme system may have been particularly high. Therefore, it might be expected that under normal dietary conditions an even smaller effect would result. In another study, children who consumed 10 sorbitol-sweetened chewing gums/day exhibited a tendency of increased numbers of *S. mutans* in plaque but not in saliva. However, only children with high baseline counts of *S. mutans* were admitted to the study and this selection may have influenced the test result [105]. A third study was carried out in dry mouth patients who were asked to rinse their mouth 10–15 times daily with a sorbitol solution for 4 weeks. Although xerostomic patients tend to have rather high level of *S. mutans* anyhow, the results indicate that frequent use of sorbitol may further increase *S. mutans* as well as sorbitol-fermenting *S. sanguis* in these subjects [114b].

Concluding Remarks in Relation to Adaptation Phenomena

Although different studies suggest that a selection for certain sorbitol-fermenting bacteria may occur after a prolonged period of frequent sorbitol exposure, there is no evidence that such adaptive changes will result in a dental plaque that metabolizes sorbitol as rapidly as sucrose. Also in relation to potential increases of *S. mutans,* there is no doubt that frequent sucrose exposure provides an ecological advantage to this aciduric and cariogenic microorganism while frequent exposure to sorbitol has hardly any clinically relevant effect. Therefore it appears that in subjects with more or less normally functioning repair mechanisms, the potential hypoacidogenic properties of sorbitol do not represent a cariogenic threat.

The experiments that have been performed in man and monkeys in order to evaluate the effect of sorbitol on plaque formation generally, lead to the conclusion that sorbitol, in comparison to an untreated control, neither increases nor inhibits the accumulation of dental plaque [100, 106]. In comparison with a sucrose treatment (positive control), lower plaque weights were found in the sorbitol group [102, 106, 113, 122].

In consideration of all these results it seems inappropriate to question the use of sorbitol as a dentally safe sugar substitute. Metabolic and ecological adaptations in dental plaque were so far observed only in xerostomic patients and under extreme experimental conditions which have no relevance for the vast majority of the consumers of sorbitol-containing sweets.

Animal Experiments with Sorbitol

Dental caries in rats shares important features with that in humans: (1) it develops on the crowns, roots and, most frequently, in the fissures of the teeth, and (2) it is dependent on the exposure to fermentable carbohydrates in the presence of an oral microflora with *S. mutans* as the most prominent cariogenic microorganism [34]. Because of these similarities, it has been attempted to rate the relative cariogenicity of different foods and food ingredients in the rat caries model. However, depending upon the precise aim of these studies and the past experimental experience of the involved research group, different modifications and methodologies have been applied and differing results have consequently been obtained. For an assessment of the relative cariogenicity of sorbitol it seems therefore appropriate to consider collectively all data that are available, rather

Table 1. Caries studies in rats with continuous administration of sorbitol

Exp.	Diet (type)	Inoculation[1]	Treatment[2] control group	Treatment[2] sorbitol group	Administration	Days	Increase or reduction of caries[3] in comparison with negative controls (starch)	Increase or reduction of caries[3] in comparison with positive controls (sucrose)	Ref.
1	natural[1]	not spec.	basal diet	basal + 10% Sor	ad lib. / ad lib.	45 / 90	-33 / -1	-50[a,b] / -47[a,b]	178
2	SSP[m]	SM	50% starch	25% starch + 25% Sor	18 meals/day	21	+99	-77[d]	129
3	SSP[m]	SM[c]	20% starch / 25% starch	20% Sor / 25% Sor	18 meals/day / 14 meals/day	72 / 72	+650 / +263	-53[a,b] / -52[a,b]	137
4	2000[f,h]	not spec.	64% starch / 64% starch / 64% starch	54% starch + 10% Sor / 44% starch + 20% Sor / 34% starch + 30% Sor	ad lib. / ad lib. / ad lib.	55 / 55 / 55	+16[a,b] / +24[a,b] / +9[a,b]	- / - / -	128
5	SSP[m]	SM	20% Suc + 5% Glu + 25% starch	20% Suc + 5% Glu + 20% starch + 5% Sor	ad lib.	62	+8[a,b]	-	130
6	semi-purified[o]	not spec.	66% Glu / 66% Suc	46% Glu + 20% Sor / 46% Suc + 20% Sor	ad lib. / ad lib.	40 / 40	- / -	+12[d] / +23[d]	179
7	semi-purified[p]	not spec.	67% starch / 67% starch	62% starch + 5% Sor / 57 starch + 10% Sor	ad lib. / ad lib.	60 / 60	+3[e] / -20[e]	- / -	125
8	MIT 300[q]	SM	67% starch	62% starch + 5% Sor[f]	ad lib.	20	+32[g] / +50[h] / +80[i]	-13[g] / -22[h] / +68[i]	133
9	MIT 300[q]	SM	62% starch + 5% Suc	62% starch + 5% Sor (fed on alternate days)	ad lib. / ad lib.	25	+24[g] / +50[h] / +63[i]	-13[g] / -10[h] / +5[i]	133

10	natural[l]	SM	basal diet	30% Sor (provided with chocolate)	ad lib.	42	+533[j]	-56[j]	131
	natural[l]	SM	basal diet	30% Sor (provided with chocolate)	18 meals/day	42	+188[j]	-47[j]	180
11	semi-purified[r]	–	16% Suc	16% Sor	ad lib.	56	–	-79[k]	

1 Rats were inoculated with *Streptococcus mutans* (SM) of serotypes c or d and with *Actinomyces viscosus* (AV).

2 Abbreviations of test compounds: sucrose (Suc), glucose (Glu), sorbitol (Sor).

3 The reduction of caries is expressed in percents of controls. Values in parentheses are increases of caries.

a T + B + C lesions.
b Mandibular molars.
c Maxillary molars.
d B lesions.
e Special scoring system.
f Experimental period preceded by a 7-day period with a 5% sucrose diet.
g Sulcal caries scores.
h Proximal caries scores.
i Buccal caries scores.
j Caries scoring according to König.
k Total number of lesions.
l Commercially available diet, composition not reported.
m Basic part: casein (18.2%), soybean protein (4.5%), cellulose (10.5%), silicium dioxide (2.7%), soybean oil (4.5%), lard (2.3%), methionine (0.09%), choline chloride (0.29%), minerals and vitamins. To obtain the final diet, 50% of the basic part is mixed with 50% of a mixture of starch and test compounds.
n Skimmed milk powder (32%), yeast (2%), Gevral® protein (2%), wheat flour (64%), test substance added at the expense of wheat flour.
o Sucrose or glucose (46%), skimmed milk powder (32%), liver powder (2%), test substance (20%).
p Casein supplemented with B-vitamins (24%), cornoil supplemented with fat-soluble vitamins (0.5%), liver powder (0.4%), mineral premix (0.4%), Cellu flour (15%), test compound(s) (67%).
q Cornstarch (62%), lactalbumin (20%), cottenseed oil (3%), cellulose (6%), vitamin premix (1%), mineral premix (3%), test compound (5%).
r Wheat starch (30%), white flour (19.75%), skimmed milk powder (32%), liver powder (2%), vitamin-mineral-essential fatty acid premix (0.25%), test substance (16%).

than to base the opinion on specific though perhaps very sophisticated studies.

The results of a number of such rat experiments are presented in table 1 and 2. Table 1 reviews the data of studies in which sorbitol was fed to the rats together with their normal diet. Table 2 contains the results of experiments in which sorbitol was intermittently fed or topically applied in order to mimic human snacking habits and in order to reduce the daily administered dose.

The results of the surveyed rat caries studies with sorbitol vary widely. Depending upon the experimental design it was found that sorbitol may be anticariogenic [123, 124], noncariogenic [125, 126], slightly cariogenic [62, 127–133], or nearly as cariogenic as sucrose [134, 135].

On balance, the presented data demonstrate that the sorbitol-treated animals exhibited in the majority of the studies somewhat higher caries scores than the starch-fed, negative controls. On the other hand, sorbitol-treated rats developed almost invariably less caries than their littermates which were exposed to sucrose (as a positive control). Overall, these results indicate that, under the conditions of the rat caries test, sorbitol is slightly but distinctly more cariogenic than native starch which is considered to be essentially noncariogenic. The data also demonstrate that the substitution of sucrose by sorbitol is normally associated with a significant decrease in caries formation. However, the view that sorbitol has an active caries-reversing effect, i.e. that it is actively combating the cariogenic attack of sucrose in the diet, is based on the results of a single study only [123]. Some supporting evidence from an older study is difficult to assess because the animals were not superinfected with *S. mutans* and because an unusual caries scoring technique was applied [124].

In principle, sorbitol may contribute to caries formation in two different ways: (1) it may serve as a fermentable, hypoacidogenic substrate for some members of the oral flora and (2) it may increase the cariogenic activity of the dental plaque by promoting the growth of *S. mutans* which is capable of utilizing sorbitol and which therefore gains a competitive advantage over other plaque organisms in the presence of sorbitol. As regards the first possibility, sorbitol exhibits a rather low acidogenicity as demonstrated also in comparative measurements of sulcal plaque pH in rats exposed to topical applications of sorbitol [136]. Not surprisingly, therefore, sorbitol was more or less noncariogenic in those studies in which the animals were not inoculated with *S. mutans* (table 1, experiments 1 and 7). On the other hand, it was found that alternate feeding of sucrose

Table 2. Experimental caries studies in rats with intermittent administration of sorbitol

Exp.	Inocu-lation[1]	Main meals all groups	Intermittent meals[2] control group	Intermittent meals[2] sorbitol group	Days	Increase or decrease of caries in sorbitol group in comparison with negative controls[3]	Increase or decrease of caries in sorbitol group in comparison with positive controls[3] (sucrose)	Ref.
1	SM[d]	20% Suc + 5% Glu (12 meals/day)	starch (6 meals/day)	33% Sor (6 meals/day)	10	-9[a,b]	-	130
2	SM[c]	20% Suc + 10% Glu (4 meals/day)	starch (14 meals/day)	25% (14 meals/day)	72	+264	-52[a,b]	137
3	SM, AV	65.5% Suc (ad lib, days 1-5)	starch (ad lib., days 6-15)	3% Sor + 3% Man		-22[g,b]	-39[g,b]	123
4	SM, AV	20% Suc (ad lib.) (ad lib.)	water (5×150 µl topical appl./day) (5×200 µl topical appl./day)	Sor (50% soln)	23 23	-30[a,b,d] -19[a,b]	-20[a,b,d] +3[a,b]	181
5	SM, AV	56% Suc (25 meals/day)	water (twice 150 µl after meals)	Sor (50% soln)	20	+91[a,b] +200[h]	-5[a,b] -22[h]	135
6	SM	MIT 200	water (3×1 ml topical appl./day)	Sor (33% soln with 0.05% saccharin)	51	+51[e]	-39[e,f]	127
7	SM	56% Suc (3 meals/day)	water (twice after each meal)	Sor (60% soln)	35	+9	-26	182
8	SM	MIT 200 (days 1-22)	0.05% asp. soln	Sor (20% soln)	42	+36[e,h]	-56[e,h]	183

[1] Rats were were inoculated with *Streptococcus mutans* (SM) of serotypes c or d and with *Actinomyces viscosus* (AV).
[2] Abbreviations of test compounds: sucrose (Suc), glucose (Glu), sorbitol (Sor), mannitol (Man).
[3] The reduction of caries is expressed in percents of controls.
[a] T + B + C lesions; [b] Mandibular molars; [c] Maxillary molars; [d] Positive control: glucose soln.; [e] Sulcal caries score; [f] Positive control: 70% Suc soln.; [g] Total lesions. ; [h] B + C lesions.

Table 3. Caries studies with sorbitol in humans[a]

Participants Initial age years	Mode of sorbitol administration (dose)	Duration of study, days	Groups	Caries increment (Δ DMFS)	Ref.
Children 11–12	tablets (dose not specified)	24	untreated sorbitol	ND[b] ND[b]	140
Children 8–12	chewing tablets (containing 1.2 g sorbitol and 45 mg calcium phosphate; 3 tablets/day)	24	untreated sorbitol	5.4[c] 5.2[c]	141
Children 3–12	chocolate (daily 20 g containing 40% sucrose or sorbitol)	36	6- to 10-year-olds sucrose sorbitol 11- to 14-years-olds sucrose sorbitol	2.89 0.71 8.90 6.89	145
Children 7–11	chewing gum (2 sticks/day)	24	no gum (controls) sorbitol gum	4.70[d] 4.63[d]	142
Children (deaf or blind, school age)	chewing gum (5 sticks/day)	30	sucrose gum sorbitol gum	5.23[d] 3.93[d]*	144
Children 7–12	chewing gum (3 sticks/day)	26	no gum sorbitol gum	5.89 5.95	143

Statistical significance: * p < 0.05.
[a] For studies on mixtures of sorbitol with xylitol, see [177, 184].
[b] DMFS values were not determined but the number of originally sound teeth becoming carious after 2 years was not significantly different between the two groups.
[c] D_2FS, only progressive lesions considered.
[d] DFS.

and sorbitol resulted in significantly higher counts of *S. mutans* than when only sucrose was administered [133], and in two other rat studies, higher plaque levels of *S. mutans* were observed in the sorbitol-treated animals than in the starch-fed controls [132, 137]. However, such effects on *S. mutans* were not seen consistently [113, 130] and corresponding investigations in humans did also give conflicting results [104, 109, 114]. Nonetheless, these observations suggest that the weak cariogenic potential of sorbitol may be related more to its effects on plaque ecology than to its low fermentability.

Although the reasons for the variance between the different rat studies and for the specific results of individual studies are far from being clear, the heterogeneity of the results indicates that utmost caution must be applied in extrapolating the animal data to humans. In this regard, a number of factors must be considered which, on the one hand, accelerate caries formation in rats and thus allow to obtain data in short periods of time but which, on the other hand, make the interpretation of the results more difficult. In this respect, particularly important factors are (1) the frequency with which the test substances and diets are consumed by the rats, and (2) the virulence and metabolic properties of the bacterial strains which are inoculated in order to render the dental plaque more cariogenic.

Considering these factors, the experimental conditions of the surveyed rat studies differ appreciably from those encountered in humans with normal dietary habits. Typically, the frequency of sorbitol exposure ranked between 5 and 18 times/day in programme-fed rats. For ad libitum fed rats an age-dependent meal frequency of about 9–14 times/day has been estimated [138, 139]. Clearly, the risk of adaptation of the oral microflora to sorbitol increases with the frequency of exposure causing both an enhanced acid production and increased levels of S. mutans in the dental plaque [97]. Thus, the cariogenicity of sorbitol is considerably higher under the conditions of the animal experiment than under normal conditions of use by man.

Another important consideration in extrapolating the animal results to humans concerns the microbiological and biochemical characteristics of the plaque flora and, in particular, of the microorganisms with which the animals are superinfected at the start of the experiment. In most studies specific strains of S. mutans were employed for this purpose. Since most strains of this bacterium effectively metabolize sorbitol, this procedure may directly influence the test results. Unfortunately, comparative data on different strains in relation to relative fermentation rates and cariogenic activity in sorbitol-fed rats are lacking, but it may safely be assumed that the practice of inoculating the test animals with S. mutans augments the cariogenic response to sorbitol.

In conclusion, it appears that the cariogenic potential of sorbitol may be overestimated if it is derived from the results of animal studies only. On the other hand, it must be recognized that the animal data at least suggest that a certain degree of cariogenicity must be suspected if sorbitol is consumed at a high frequency by individuals who harbour high numbers of cariogenic microorganisms in dental plaque.

Caries Studies with Sorbitol in Humans

The cariogenicity of sorbitol and its dental benefits as a sugar substitute have been tested in different long-term trials in school-age children (table 3). In a first study that was conducted 25 years ago, sorbitol-based tablets were tested in school-age children. After 1 year of treatment, significantly fewer molar teeth developed new caries in the sorbitol-treated group than in the untreated control group. However, no corresponding differences could be observed in molars, nor in all other teeth at termination of the study after 2 years [140]. While the results of this first study might be questioned because of a probably poor compliance of the participants (35% of the children disliked the test product), essentially identical observations were made in a subsequent study with sorbitol-sweetened chewing tablets [141]. Again the greatest difference between the sorbitol-treated children and an untreated control group was found on the occlusal surfaces of the maxillary first molar. During the 2-year study period, 25.1% of the originally sound surfaces became carious in the controls while in the sorbitol group, only 15.7% of the surfaces were affected by caries. However, despite this obvious effect on molar teeth, only a relatively small (approx. 10%) difference was found if total DFS increments were compared. While the authors concluded that the observed, statistically significant reduction in caries may be of little practical relevance, the data certainly indicate that the regular consumption of sorbitol-sweetened chewables did not promote caries formation. An identical conclusion was reached by the authors of two other studies in which school children consumed 2–3 sorbitol chewing gums daily for a period of about 2 years [142, 143].

A principally different, but in terms of practical relevance perhaps more appropriate design, was chosen in two futher studies in which a sucrose-treated, i.e. positive control group was compared with a sorbitol-treated test group. In one study, chewing gum was used as the vehicle, in the other chocolate was provided to the children [144, 145]. From the results of both studies it appears that the use of sorbitol as a sugar substitute may provide benefits in terms of caries prevention as the caries increment was reduced by about 25 and 40% in the sorbitol groups of the chewing gum and chocolate study, respectively. That this 'reduction' resulted probably from an increased caries challenge in the sucrose-treated controls rather than from an active caries-inhibiting effect of sorbitol is largely irrelevant from a public health point of view.

In none of the mentioned long-term studies was evidence for a direct or indirect cariogenicity of sorbitol observed. Although bacterial adaptation phenomena had not been examined specifically in these trials, it appears therefore that, in a normal healthy population, such effects have little relevance in terms of caries formation. Reports from other investigations seem to support this conclusion [121].

Potential Cariostatic Properties of Sugar Substitutes

Definition and Principal Mechanisms

The formation of caries is a dynamic process which, in its initial phase, is reversible to some extent [146–149]. The balance between caries progression, i.e. demineralization of the tooth enamel, and caries regression, i.e. remineralization of incipient lesions, is influenced by the interplay of different exogenous and endogenous factors. While certain exogenous factors such as the presence of an acidogenic and aciduric dental plaque together with an abundant and frequent supply of easy fermentable carbohydrates favour the demineralization of the enamel, there exist on the other hand endogenous protective factors which counteract this destructive process. Among these natural defense systems, salivary remineralization is considered to be the most important reparative mechanism against tooth decay [150, 151]. Other defense mechanisms include the salivary lactoperoxidase system, lysozyme, lactoferrin and secretory antibodies which are directed against the bacterial colonization of the oral surfaces in a more or less specific way.

Agents which induce shifts in the oral environment from conditions that predispose to caries to those which tend to slow down caries progression, are considered to exert a cariostatic effect. The mechanisms through which cariostatic agents as, for example, fluorides, antimicrobials and mineral salts mediate such shifts are manifold and include effects on the mineral phase of the tooth enamel, changes of the metabolic activity and microbiological composition of dental plaque, enhancement of salivary antibacterial and remineralizing factors, as well as combinations of these effects.

Several investigators have proposed that certain food ingredients and food additives may have an active role in decreasing the risk of enamel demineralization or, conversely, of enhancing remineralization. Examples include calcium glycerophosphate [152], sodium phytate [153], calcium sucrose phosphate [154], calcium lactate [155], glycerol monolaurin [156], as well as different sugar substitutes [157] and intense sweeteners [158]. Sweeteners may interact with various caries-promoting and caries-inhibiting factors in several ways. By stimulating salivary flow they improve the clearance of carbohydrate residues from the oral cavity, they neutralize dental plaque, and they promote the remineralization of incipient lesions. Furthermore, beneficial changes of plaque ecology and metabolism may result indirectly from the absence of sucrose and directly from specific inhibitory metabolic effects.

Salivation-Mediated Effects

An increase of the salivary flow rate is the physiological response to the ingestion of foods. Sweet-, sour- or bitter-tasting products elicit a particularly strong response. Mastication of a food further enhances salivation. Consumption of a sweet chewing gum leads, therefore, to a near maximum stimulation of the salivary flow rate [159]. This response has different beneficial sequelae.

First, an increased salivary flow accelerates the clearance of the oral cavity from residual fermentable components of previously ingested foods. This process seems to be very effective as it has been found that the chewing of a sugar-free gum with sorbitol or xylitol clears the oral cavity from a preceding glucose challenge more efficiently than tooth-brushing [160].

Second, saliva exerts an important neutralizing action on dental plaque. Because of its considerable buffer capacity, saliva corrects pH changes of the dental plaque caused by the fermentation of sugars [161, 162]. Telemetric recordings of plaque pH values after a sucrose challenge followed by the consumption of a sugar-free, e.g. sorbitol-sweetened gum have demonstrated this effect convincingly [163–165].

Third, saliva has a remineralization potential residing in its supersaturation with regard to calcium phosphate [166]. During periods with increased salivary flow, higher amounts of calcium and phosphate are available for redeposition in partly demineralized tooth enamel. However, an incorporation of calcium phosphate on the tooth surface and a formation of apatite-like solid structures occurs only if the pH is sufficiently high, and if it is maintained at such level for a sufficient period of time.

This latter condition is not met after consumption of sucrose-based sweets. In this case, the acid formation in dental plaque completely offsets the beneficial effect of the salivary stimulation. If, on the other hand, saliva is stimulated by sugar-free sweets, the increased salivary flow may fully support remineralization. The practical relevance of this process has been documented in an in vivo experiment in which intraoral sucrose-induced demineralization was efficiently inhibited by sorbitol chewing gum, as well as by a study in which extensive remineralization of artificial white spots was observed if Lycasin®-sweetened candies were consumed at a high frequency for a 2-week period [167]. This finding confirms and extends corresponding results from a study in rats, in which the feeding of various sweeteners also promoted the remineralization of demineralized defects [123, 168].

Effects on Dental Plaque
In the oral cavity there is a shortage of bacterial nutrients most of the time. Consequently, the frequency and duration for which oral bacteria are exposed to easy fermentable carbohydrates has a profound effect on the composition and metabolic activity of the dental plaque. A frequent exposure to sucrose and other carbohydrates results in a frequent acidification of the plaque which favours the growth of aciduric, i.e. acid-tolerant bacteria such as lactobacilli and *S. mutans* [169, 170]. In addition, the exposure to sucrose supports the formation of extracellular polysaccharides which play an important role as structural polymers in the accumulation and cohesion of dental plaque. Furthermore, intracellular polysaccharides may be synthesized by many bacteria when sugars are present in excess. During periods when no sugars are supplied, these polymers will be used as an energy source, and acids are formed again as metabolic end products. All these sugar-mediated changes are obviously undesirable because they increase the cariogenicity of the dental plaque [171]. Conversely, a less aciduric, acidogenic and therefore cariogenic plaque develops if sorbitol is used in place of sucrose [86]. The reason for this is that plaque acidification is minimal after exposure to sorbitol [165, 172] and that sorbitol does not promote plaque formation and adhesion by insoluble glucan synthesis [68].

While xylitol exerts under certain conditions a direct inhibitory action on the growth and metabolism of certain oral bacteria, no corresponding effects have been observed for sorbitol. However, it has recently been reported that sorbitol may enhance the inhibitory potential of xylitol on the growth of *S. mutans* [173]. Since it is also known that xylitol inhibits the fermentation of sorbitol by *S. mutans* [174–176] mixtures of sorbitol and xylitol may have superior properties than sorbitol alone. In this regard, it is noteworthy that chewing gums sweetened with a xylitol/sorbitol mixture decreased plaque formation to a similar extent as gums sweetened with xylitol only [107]. In another study, less plaque was formed during 4 days' consumption of a xylitol- or sorbitol/xylitol-sweetened gum than during a corresponding period with consumption of sorbitol-sweetened gums [108].

Relevance of Cariostatic Properties in Terms of Caries Prevention

The practical relevance of the mentioned cariostatic mechanisms can only be determined from the results of long-term caries studies in man. As may be seen from the data summarized in table 3, a significant reduction of caries increments was observed only in those studies in which the sorbitol group was compared with a sucrose-treated control group. In comparison to untreated controls, no decrease in caries increments was observed that would suggest the action of cariostatic effects. However, more promising results were reported recently from a caries study in which children received xylitol/sorbitol-sweetened gums over a period of 2 years. The observed reduction of caries increment by 60% suggests that such combinations may be more effective than sorbitol alone [177].

Conclusion

Sorbitol is a commonly used sweetener in sugar-free confectionery, in special dietetic products for diabetics, and in sugar-free medicines. Because of its humectant properties, it is applied in toothpaste as well as in certain food products.

The cariogenicity of sorbitol has been evaluated in numerous studies in vitro and in vivo. Experiments with isolated oral microorganisms and dental plaque, as well as plaque pH investigations have been carried out in order to determine the fermentability and acidogenicity of sorbitol under different conditions. The assessment of its cariogenic potential includes numerous studies with rats as well as a few long-term caries trials in humans.

Taken collectively, the data indicate that, under normal conditions of use, the acidogenicity of sorbitol is negligibly small and that it is virtually noncariogenic. However, sorbitol does not possess specific cariostatic properties. Although there are some data showing that frequent consumption of sorbitol may result in a marginally increased acid production in dental plaque, and perhaps in slightly increased numbers of sorbitol-fermenting, cariogenic microorganisms such as *S. mutans* and lactobacilli, it does not appear justified to generally question its use as a dentally safe bulk sugar substitute for sugar-free sweets.

References

1   Sreebny, L.M.: Sugar and human dental caries. World Rev. Nutr. Diet. *40:* 19–65 (1982).
2   Newbrun, E.: Sugar and dental caries: a review of human studies. Science *217:* 418–423 (1982).
3   Sheiham, A.: Sugars and dental decay. Lancet *i:* 282–284 (1983).
4   Rugg-Gunn, A.J.: Diet and dental caries; in Murray, J.J. (ed.): The Prevention of Dental Disease, pp. 3–82 (Oxford University Press, Oxford 1983).
5   Rugg-Gunn, A.J.; Hackett, A.F.; Appleton, D.R.; Jenkins, G.N.; Eastone, J.E.: Relationship between dietary habits and caries increment assessed over two years in 405 English adolescent school children. Arch. Oral Biol. *29:* 983–992 (1984).
6   Newbrun, E.: Epidemiology of caries – worldwide. Dtsch. Zahnärztl. Z. *42:* S8–S15 (1987).
7   Klimek, J.; Rauch, P.; Hellwig, E.; Prinz, H.: Ernährungsgewohnheiten, Zahnkaries und Mundhygiene bei 7-jährigen Schulkindern. Annual Report of Deutsche Gesellschaft für Zahnerhaltung e.V., Berlin 1987.
8   Burt, B.A.; Eklund, S.A.; Morgan, K.J.; Larkin, F.E.; Guire, K.E.; Brown, L.O.; Weintraub, J.A.: The effects of sugars intake and frequency of ingestion on dental caries increment in a three-year longitudinal study. J. Dent. Res. *67:* 1422–1429 (1988).
9   Sundin, B.; Birkhed, D.; Granath, L.: Is there not a strong relationship nowadays between caries and consumption of sweets? Swed. Dent. J. *7:* 103–108 (1983).
10 Koch, G.: Evidence for declining caries prevalence in Sweden. J. Dent. Res. *61:* 1340–1345 (1982).
11 Bille, J.; Hesselgren, K.; Thylstrup, A.: Dental caries in Danish 7-, 11- and 13-year-old children in 1963, 1972 and 1981. Caries Res. *20:* 534–542 (1986).
12 Burton, V.J.; Rob, M.I.; Craig, G.G.; Lawson, J.S.: Changes in the caries experience of 12-year-old Sydney school children between 1963 and 1982. Med. J. Aust. *140:* 405–407 (1984).
13 Holt, R.D.; Bulman, S.: A third study of caries in pre-school children in Camden (abstract). J. Dent. Res. *66:* 898 (1987).
14 Naujoks, R.: Epidemiologie der Zahnkaries in der Bundesrepublik Deutschland. Dtsch. Zahnärztl. Z. *42:* S16–S19 (1987).
15 Tervonen, T.; Ainamo, J.: Constant proportion of decayed teeth in adults aged 25, 35, 50 and 65 years in a high-caries area. Caries Res. *22:* 45–49 (1988).

16 Glass, R.L.; Alman, J.E.; Chauncey, H.H.: A 10-year longitudinal study of caries incidence rates in a sample of male adults in the USA. Caries Res. *21:* 360–367 (1987).

17 Burt, B.A.: The future of the caries decline. J. Public Health Dent. *45:* 261–269 (1985).

18 Birkhed, D.; Sundin, B.; Westin, S.: Per capita consumption of sugar-containing products and dental caries in Sweden from 1960 to 1985. Community Dent. Oral Epidemiol. *17:* 41–43 (1989).

19 Penttilä, P.-L.; Salminen, S.; Niemi, E.: Estimates on the intake of food additives in Finland. Z. Lebensmittelunters. Forsch. *186:* 11–15 (1988).

20 Mäkinen, K.K.; Söderling, E.: A quantitative study of mannitol, sorbitol, xylitol, and xylose in wild berries and commercial fruits. J. Food Sci. *45:* 367–374 (1980).

21 Weiss, J.; Sämann, H.: Ergebnisse von Untersuchungen über die *D*-Sorbitgehalte von Fruchtsäften. Mitt. Klosterneuburg *29:* 81–84 (1979).

22 Pitkänen, E.: The serum polyol pattern and the urinary polyol excretion in diabetic and uremic patients. Clin. Chim. Acta *38:* 221–230 (1972).

23 Servo, C., et al: Gas chromatographic separation and mass spectrometric identification of polyols in human cerebrospinal fluid and plasma. Acta Neurol. Scand. *56:* 104–110 (1977).

24 Lauwers, A.-M.; Daumerie, C.; Henquin, J.C.: Intestinal absorption of sorbitol and effects of its acute administration on glucose homeostasis in normal rats. Br. J. Nutr. *53:* 53–62 (1985).

25 Sener, A.; Hutton, J.C.; Schoonveydt, J.; Tinant, A.; Urbain, M.; Malaisse, W.J.: Relationship of endogenous to dietary sorbitol. A study in normal and diabetic rats. Diabète Metab. *5:* 217–222 (1979).

26 Grossklaus, R.; Klingebiel, L.; Lorenz, S.; Pahlke, G.: Risk-benefit analyses of new sugar substitutes. 2. The formation of short-chain fatty acids in the ceca of nonadapted and adapted juvenile rats. Nutr. Res. *4:* 459–468 (1984).

27 FAO/WHO Expert Committee on Food Additives: Evaluation of certain food additives and contaminants (26th report). WHO Tech. Rep. Ser. No. 683 (1982).

28 Life Sciences Research Office: Dietary sugars in health and disease. III. Sorbitol – Report prepared for the Center for Food Safety and Applied Nutrition, Food and Drug Administration, Washington, D.C., under contract No. FDA 223-75-2090 by the Life Sciences Research Office, Federation of American Societies for Experimental Biology (FASEB), Bethesda, Md., 1979, p. 85.

29 Life Sciences Research Office: Health aspects of sugar alcohols and lactose. Report prepared for the Center for Food Safety and Applied Nutrition, Food and Drug Administration, Washington, D.C., under contract No. FDA 223-83-2020 by the Life Sciences Research Office, Federation of American Societies for Experimental Biology (FASEB), Bethesda, Md. 1986, p. 85.

30 Förster, H.; Mehnert, H.: Die orale Anwendung von Sorbit als Zuckeraustauschstoff in der Diät des Diabetes mellitus. Aktuel. Ernähr. *5:* 245–257 (1979).

31 MacDonald, J.; Keyser, A.; Pacy, D.: Some effects, in man, of varying the load of glucose, sucrose, fructose or sorbitol on various metabolites in blood. Am. J. Clin. Nutr. *31:* 1305–1311 (1978).

32 Stephan, R.M.: Changes in hydrogen-ion concentration on tooth surfaces and in carious lesions. J. Am. Dent. Assoc. *27:* 718 (1940).

33   Imfeld, T.: Identification of low caries risk dietary components; in Monographs in
     Oral Science, vol. 11, pp. 1–198. (Karger, Basel 1983).
34   Tanzer, J.M.: Testing food cariogenicity with experimental animals. J. Dent. Res.
     65: spec. issue, pp. 1491–1497 (1986).
35   Clarkson, B.H.: In vitro methods for testing the cariogenic potential of foods. J.
     Dent. Res. 65: spec. issue, pp. 1516–1519 (1986).
36   Platt, D.; Werrin, S.R.: Acid production from alditols by oral streptococci. J. Dent.
     Res. 58: 1733–1734 (1979).
37   Shockley, T.E.; Randless, C.I.; Dodd, M.C.: The fermentation of sorbitol by certain
     acidogenic oral microorganisms. J. Dent. Res. 35: 233–244 (1956).
38   Gehring, F.: Zum Sorbitabbau durch Streptokokken unter besonderer Berücksichti-
     gung der Mundflora. Dtsch. Zahnärztl. Z. 23: 810–819 (1968).
39   Gehring, F.: Saccharose und Zuckeraustauschstoffe im mikrobiologischen Test.
     Dtsch. Zahärztl. Z. 26: 1162–1171 (1971).
40   Grubb, T.C.: Studies on the fermentation of sorbitol by oral microorganisms. J.
     Dent. Res. 24: 31–44 (1945).
41   Crowley, M.C.; Harner, V.; Bennett, A.S.; Jay, P.H.: Comparative fermentability of
     sorbitol, glucose and glycerol by common oral microorganisms. J. Am. Dent. Assoc.
     52: 148–154 (1956).
42   Carlsson, J.: A numerical taxonomic study of human oral streptococci. Odont. Revy
     19: 137–160 (1968).
43   Edwardsson, S.: Characteristics of caries-inducing human streptococci resembling
     Streptococcus mutans. Arch. Oral Biol. 13: 637–646 (1968).
44   Guggenheim, B.: Microbiology of dental plaque with special reference to streptococ-
     ci. Caries Res. 2: 147–163 (1968).
45   Deibel, R.H.; Seeley, H.W.: Gram-positive cocci. Family II. Streptococceae; in
     Buchanan, R.E.; Gibbons, N.E. (eds): Bergey's Manual of Determinative Bacterio-
     logy; 8th ed., pp. 490–509 (Williams & Wilkins, Baltimore 1974).
46   Edwardsson, S.: Bacteriological studies on deep areas of carious dentine. Odont.
     Revy 25: suppl. 32 (1974).
47   Shklair, I.L.; Keene, H.J.: A biochemical scheme for the separation of the five vari-
     eties of Streptococcus mutans. Arch. Oral Biol. 19: 1079–1081 (1974).
48   Edwardsson, S.; Birkhed, D.; Mejàre, B.: Acid production from Lycasin®, maltitol,
     sorbitol and xylitol by oral streptococci and lactobacilli. Acta Odontol. Scand. 35:
     257–263 (1977).
49   Soyer, C.; Frank, R.M.: Influence du milieu de culture sur la croissance du Strepto-
     coccus mutans ATTCC 25175 en présence de différents glucides et leurs dérivés. J.
     Biol. Buccale 7: 295–301 (1979).
50   Gallagher, J.H.C.; Pearce, E.J.F.: The fermentation of sucrose, sorbitol, and xylitol
     by Propionibacterium avidum, resulting in the formation of caries-like lesions in
     animal. N.Z. Dent. J. 79: 75–79 (1983).
51   Mejàre, B.; Edwardsson, S.: Streptococcus milleri (Guthof), an indigenous organism
     of the human oral cavity. Arch. Oral Biol. 20: 755–762 (1975).
52   Havenaar, R.; Huis In't Veld, J.H.J.; Backer-Dirks, O.; De Stoppelaar, J.D.: Some
     bacteriological aspects of sugar substitutes; in Guggenheim, B. (ed.): Health and
     Sugar Substitutes. Proc. ERGOB Conf., Geneva 1978, pp. 192–198 (Karger, Basel
     1978).

53 Brown, A.T.; Wittenberger, C.L.: Mannitol and sorbitol catabolism in *Streptococcus mutans*. Arch. Oral Biol. *18:* 117–126 (1973).

54 Maryanski, J.H.; Wittenberger, C.L.: Mannitol transport in *Streptococcus mutans*. J. Bacteriol. *124:* 1475–1481 (1975).

55 Slee, A.M.; Tanzer, J.M.: The repressible metabolism of sorbitol (*D*-glucitol) by intact cells of the oral plaque-forming bacterium *Streptococcus mutans*. Arch. Oral Biol. *28:* 839–845 (1983).

56 Dallmeier, E.; Bestmann, H.-J.; Kröncke, A.: Über den Abbau von Glukose und Sorbit durch Plaque-Streptokokken. Dtsch. Zahnärztl. Z. *25:* 887–898 (1970).

57 Yamada, T.; Takahashi-Abbe, S.; Abbe, K.: Effects of oxygen on pyruvate formate-lyase in situ and sugar metabolism of *Streptococcus mutans* and *Streptococcus sanguis*. Infect. Immun. *47:* 129–134 (1985).

58 Takahashi, N.; Abbe, K.; Takahashi-Abbe, S.; Yamada, T.: Oxygen sensitivity of sugar metabolism and interconversion of pyruvate formate-lyase in intact cells of *Streptococcus mutans* and *Streptococcus sanguis*. Infect. Immun. *55:* 652–656 (1987).

59 Svensäter, G.; Takahashi-Abbe, S.; Abbe, K.; Birkhed, D.; Yamada, T.; Edwardsson, S.: Anaerobic and aerobic metabolism of sorbitol in *Streptococcus sanguis* and *Streptococcus mitior*. J. Dent. Res. *64:* 1286–1289 (1985).

60 Kalfas, S.; Birkhed, D.: Effect of aerobic and anaerobic atmosphere on acid production from sorbitol in suspensions of dental plaque and oral streptococci. Caries Res. *20:* 237–243 (1986).

61 Gehring, F.: Über die Säurebildung kariesätiologisch wichtiger Streptokokken aus Zuckern und Zuckeralkoholen unter besonderer Berücksichtigung von Isomaltit und Isomaltulose. Z. Ernährungswiss., suppl. 15: 16–27 (1973).

62 Gehring, F.; Karle, E.J.: Der Saccharoseaustauschstoff Palatinit® unter besonderer Berücksichtigung mikrobiologischer und kariesprophylaktischer Aspekte. Z. Ernährungswiss. *20:* 96–106 (1981).

63 Drucker, D.B.; Verran, J.: Comparative effects of the substance-sweeteners glucose, sorbitol, sucrose, xylitol and trichlorosucrose on lowering of pH by two oral *Streptococcus mutans* strains in vitro. Arch. Oral Biol. *24:* 965–970 (1980).

64 Yamamoto, H.; Kawanishi, S.; Maki, Y.; Matsukubo, T.; Takaesu, Y.: Evaluation of acidogenicity of various sugar substitutes using *S. mutans*. J. Dent. Res. *66:* 301, abstr. 1557 (1987).

65 Westergren, G.; Krasse, B.; Birkhed, D.; Edwardsson, S.: Genetic transfer of markers for sorbitol (*D*-glucitol) metabolism in oral streptococci. Archs. Oral Biol. *26:* 403–407 (1981).

66a Stegmeier, K.; Dallmeier, E.; Bestmann, H.-J.; Kröncke, A.: Untersuchungen über den Sorbitabbau unter Verwendung von C-markierten Substanzen und Gaschromatographie. Dtsch. Zahnärztl. Z. *26:* 1129–1134 (1971).

66b Kalfas, S.; Maki, Y.; Birkhed, D.; Edwardsson, S.: Effect of pH on acid production from sorbitol in washed cell suspensions of oral bacteria. Caries Res. *24:* 107–112 (1990).

67 Lounatmaa, K.; Tuompo, H.; Meurman, J.H.: Biochemistry and ultrastructure of the *Streptococcus mutans* cell wall after various carbon sources. J. Dent. Res. *60:* 250, abstr. 27 (1981).

68 Imai, S.; Takeuchi, K.; Shibata, S.; Yoshikawa, S.; Kitahata, S.; Okada, S.; Araya, S.;

Nisizawa, T.: Screening of sugars inhibitory against sucrose-dependent synthesis and adherence of insoluble glucan and acid production by *Streptococcus mutans.* J. Dent. Res. *63:* 1293–1297 (1984).

69   Söderling, E.; Alaraeisänen, L.; Scheinin, A.; Mäkinen, K.K.: Effect of xylitol and sorbitol on polysaccharide production by and adhesive properties of *Streptococcus mutans.* Caries Res. *21:* 109–116 (1987).

70   Gülzow, H.-J.: Über den Abbau von Sorbit durch Plaque-Mikroorganismen. Dtsch. Zahnärztl. Z. *23:* 326–330 (1968).

71   Gülzow, H.-J.: Vergleichende Untersuchungen über den Abbau von Xylit im menschlichen Speichel. Dtsch. Zahnärztl. Z. *29:* 772–775 (1974).

72   Gülzow, H.-J.: Über den anaeroben Umsatz von Palatinit® durch Mikroorganismen der menschlichen Mundhöhle. Dtsch. Zahnärztl. Z. *37:* 669–672 (1982).

73   Mäkinen, K.K.: Microbial growth and metabolism in plaque in the presence of sugar alcohols; in Stiles, H.M.; Loesche, W.J.; O'Brien, T.C. (eds): Microbial Aspects of Dental Caries. Microbiol. Abstr. *2:* spec. supp., pp. 521–538 (1976).

74   Birkhed, D.; Edwardsson, B.; Svensson, B.; Moskovitz, F.; Frostell, G.: Acid production from sorbitol in human dental plaque. Arch. Oral Biol. *23:* 971–975 (1978).

75   Hayes, M.L.; Roberts, K.R.: The breakdown of glucose, xylitol and other sugar alcohols by human dental plaque bacteria. Arch. Oral Biol. *23:* 445–451 (1978).

76   Birkhed, D.: Automatic titration method for determination of acid production from sugars and sugar alcohols in small samples of dental plaque material. Caries Res. *12:* 128–136 (1978).

77   Brown, J.P.; Huang, C.T.; Oldershaw, M.D.; Bibby, B.G.: Continuous measurement of plaque pH in vitro. J. Dent. Res. *60:* 724 (1981).

78   Maki, Y.; Ohta, K.; Takazoe, I.; Matsukubo, Y.; Takaesu, Y.; Topitsoglou, V.; Frostell, G.: Acid production from isomaltulose, sucrose, sorbitol, and xylitol in suspensions of human dental plaque. Caries Res. *17:* 335–339 (1983).

79   Strübig, W.: Über den Abbau von Zucker und Zuckeraustauschstoffen durch die Mischflora der menschlichen Mundhöhle. Habilitationsschriften der Zahn-, Mund- und Kieferheilkunde (Quintessenz, Berlin 1986).

80   Igarashi, K.; Lee, I.K.; Schachtele, C.F.: Comparison of in vivo human dental plaque pH changes within artificial fissures and at interproximal sites. Caries Res. *23:* 417–422 (1989).

81   Fosdick, L.S.; Englander, H.R.; Hoerman, K.C.; Kesel, R.G.: A comparison of pH values of in vivo dental plaque after sucrose and sorbitol mouth rinses. J. Am. Dent. Assoc. *55:* 191–195 (1957).

82   Frostell, G.: Dental plaque pH in relation to intake of carbohydrate products. Acta Odontol. Scand. *27:* 3–29 (1969).

83   Frostell, G.: Effects of mouth rinses with sucrose, glucose, fructose, lactose, sorbitol and Lycasin® on the pH of dental plaque. Odont. Revy *24:* 217–226 (1973).

84   Rugg-Gunn, A.J.: Effect of Lycasin® upon plaque pH when taken as a syrup or as a boiled sweet. Caries Res. *22:* 375–376 (1988).

85   Kleber, C.J.; Schimmele, R.G.; Putt, M.S.; Muhler, J.C.: The effect of tablets composed of various mixtures, sugar alcohols and sugars upon plaque pH in children. J. Dent. Res. *58:* 614–618 (1979).

86   Graber, T.M.; Muller, T.P.; Bhatia, V.D.: The effect of xylitol gum and rinses on plaque acidogenesis in patients with fixed orthodontic appliances. Swed. Dent. J. *15:* suppl., pp. 41–55 (1982).

87 Rugg-Gunn, A.J.; Edgar, W.M.; Jenkins, G.N.: The effect of eating some British snacks upon the pH of human dental plaque. Br. Dent. J. *145:* 95–100 (1978).

88 Vratsanos, S.M.; Mandel, I.D.: The effect of sucrose and hexitol containing chewing gums on plaque acidogenesis in vivo. Pharmacol. Therapeut. Dent. *6:* 87–91 (1981).

89 Zuccato, E.; Andreoletti, M.; Mussini, E.; Conca, R.; Ferrara, A.; Pecchioni, A.: Produzione di H_2 e CH_4 come espressione dinamica del metabolismo batterico nell'ecosistema orale. Mondo Odostom *4:* 25–30 (1986).

90 Imfeld, T.: Evaluation of the cariogenicity of confectionery by intra-oral wire-telemetry. Helv. Odontol. Acta *21:* 1–28 (1977).

91 Neff, D.: Acid production from different carbohydrate sources in human plaque in situ. Caries Res. *1:* 78–87 (1967).

92 Mühlemann, H.R.; De Boever, J.: Radiotelemetry of the pH of interdental areas exposed to various carbohydrates; in McHugh, W.D. (ed.): Dental Plaque (Thomson, Dundee 1969).

93 Schneider, P.H.; Mühlemann, H.R.: Zuckerfreie zahnschonende Kaugummis und Bonbons. Schweiz. Monatsschr. Zahnheilkd. *86:* 150–166 (1976).

94 Linke, H.A.B.: Sugar alcohols and dental health. World Rev. Nutr. Diet. *47:* 134–162 (1986).

95 Abbe, K.; Takahashi, S.; Yamada, T.: Involvement of oxygen-sensitive pyruvate formate-lyase in mixed-acid fermentation by *Streptococcus mutans* under strictly anaerobic conditions. J. Bacteriol. *152:* 175–182 (1982).

96 Birkhed, D.; Edwardsson, S.; Kalfas, S.; Svensäter, G.: Cariogenicity of sorbitol. Swed. Dent. J. *8:* 147–154 (1984).

97 Birkhed, D.; Svensäter, G.; Kalfas, S.; Edwardsson, S.: The risk of adaptation of the oral microflora to sorbitol. Dtsch. Zahnärztl. Z. *42:* S141–S144 (1987).

98 Linke, H.A.B.; Castle, M.: Isolation of acid producing sorbitol-adapted bacteria from dental plaque using selective agar media. Microbios *61:* 39–48 (1990).

99 Birkhed, D.; Edwardsson, S.; Ahldén, M.-L.; Frostell, G.: Effects of 3 months' frequent consumption of hydrogenated starch hydrolysate (Lycasin®), maltitol, sorbitol and xylitol on human dental plaque. Acta Odontol. Scand. *37:* 103–115 (1979).

100 Birkhed, D.; Edwardsson, S.; Wikesjö, U.; Ahldén, M.-L.; Ainamo, J.: Effect of 4 days' consumption of chewing gum containing sorbitol or a mixture of sorbitol and xylitol on dental plaque and saliva. Caries Res. *17:* 76–88 (1983).

101 Harjola, U.; Liesmaa, H.: Effects of polyol and sucrose candies on plaque, gingivitis and lactobacillus index scores. Acta Odontol. Scand. *36:* 237–242 (1978).

102 Ainamo, J.; Sjöblom, M.; Ainamo, A.; Tiainen, L.: Growth of plaque while chewing sucrose and sorbitol flavoured gum. J. Clin. Periodontol. *4:* 151–160 (1977).

103 Ainamo, J.; Asikainen, S.; Ainamo, A.; Lathinen, A.; Sjöblom, M.: Plaque growth while chewing sorbitol and xylitol simultaneously with sucrose-flavored gum. J. Clin. Periodontol. *6:* 397–406 (1979).

104 Loesche, W.J.: The effect of sugar alcohols on plaque and saliva level of *Streptococcus mutans.* Swed. Dent. J. *8:* 125–135 (1984).

105 Loesche, W.J.; Earnest, R.; Grossman, N.S.; Corpron, R.: The effect of chewing xylitol gum on the plaque and saliva levels of *Streptococcus mutans.* J. Am. Dent. Assoc. *108:* 587–592 (1984).

106 Rateitschak-Plüss, E.M.; Guggenheim, B.: Effects of a carbohydrate-free diet and sugar substitutes on dental plaque accumulation. J. Clin. Periodontol. *9:* 239–251 (1982).

107 Söderling, E.; Mäkinen, K.K.; Chen, C.-Y.; Pape, H.R.; Loesche, W.; Mäkinen, P.-L.: Effect of sorbitol, xylitol or xylitol/sorbitol chewing gum on dental plaque. Caries Res. *23:* 378–384 (1989).

108 Topitsoglou, V.; Birkhed, D.; Larsson, L.-A.; Frostell, G.: Effect of chewing gums containing xylitol, sorbitol or a mixture of xylitol and sorbitol on plaque formation, pH changes and acid production in human dental plaque. Caries Res. *17:* 369–378 (1983).

109 Wennerholm, K.; Emilson, C.G.: Effect of frequent use of sorbitol-containing nicotine chewing gum on salivary microflora, saliva and oral sugar clearance. J. Dent. Res. *64:* 756, abstr. 9 (1985).

110 Möller, I.J.; Poulsen, S.: The effect of sorbitol-containing chewing gum on the incidence of dental caries: plaque and gingivitis in Danish schoolchildren. Community Dent. Oral Epidemiol. *1:* 58–67 (1973).

111 Rekola, M.: A comparison of the effect of xylitol and sorbitol-sweetened chewing gums on dental plaque. Proc. Finn. Dent. Soc. *78:* 128–133 (1982).

112 Mäkinen, K.K.; Virtanen, K.K.: Effect of 4.5-year use of xylitol and sorbitol on plaque. J. Dent. Res. *57:* 441–446 (1978).

113 Cornick, D.E.R.; Bowen, W.H.: The effect of sorbitol on the microbiology of the dental plaque in monkeys. Arch. Oral Biol. *17:* 1637–1648 (1972).

114a Kalfas, S.; Svensäter, G.; Birkhed, D.; Edwardsson, S.: Sorbitol adaptation of dental plaque in people with low and normal salivary-secretion rates. J. Dent. Res. *69:* 442–446 (1990).

114b Kalfas, S.; Edwardsson, S.: Sorbitol-fermenting predominant cultivable flora of human dental plaque in relation to sorbitol adaptation and salivary secretion rate. Oral Microbiol. Immunol. *5:* 33–38 (1990).

115 Kary, H.: Vergleichende Warburg-Versuche über den Abbau von Sorbit durch Mikroorganismen des Nüchternspeichels von Diabetikern und Nicht-Diabetikern; Diss. Hamburg (1986).

116 Silver, J.G.; Krasse, B.: Treatment of dental caries monitored by microbial methods: report of two cases. J. Can. Dent. Assoc. *3:* 211–215 (1985).

117 Linke, H.A.B.; Siebert, G.; Ziesenitz, S.C.: Acid production and sugar transport of sorbitol-adapted streptococci isolated from sorbitol-conditioned dental plaque. Caries Res. *23:* 96, abstr. 17 (1989).

118 Jenkins, G.N.: Salivary effects on plaque pH; in Kleinberg, I.; Ellison, S.A.; Mandel, I.D. (eds.): Proceedings Saliva and Dental Caries. Microbiol. Abstr., spec. suppl. *1:* p. 307 (1979).

119 Dreizen, S.; Brown, L.R.: Xerostomia and dental caries; in Stiles, H.M.; Loesche, W.J.; O'Brien, T.C. (eds): Proceedings Microbial Aspects of Dental Caries. Microbiol. Abstr. *1:* spec. suppl., pp. 263–273 (1976).

120 Banoczy, J.; Gabris, K.; Orosz, M.: Salivary lactobacillus counts after prolonged use of sorbit. Fogorv. Sz. *71:* 33–36 (1978).

121 Birkhed, D.; Svensäter, G.; Edwardsson, S.: Cariological studies of individuals with long-term sorbitol consumption. Caries Res. *24:* 220–223 (1990).

122 Pinter, A.; Schuder, L.; Banoczy, J.: Vergleichende Untersuchungen der belagbil-

denden Wirkung von Sorbit und Saccharose enthaltender Schokolade. Dtsch. Zahnärztl. Z. *33:* 418–420 (1978).

123 Leach, S.A.; Green, R.M.: Reversal of fissure caries in the albino rat by sweetening
agents. Caries Res. *15:* 508–511 (1981).

124 Grunberg, E.; Beskid, G.; Brin, M.: Xylitol and dental caries. Efficacy of xylitol in
reducing dental caries in rats. Int. J. Vitam. Nutr. Res. *43:* 227–232 (1973).

125 Shaw, J.H.: Inability of low levels of sorbitol and mannitol to support caries activity
in rats. J. Dent. Res. *55:* 376–382 (1976).

126 Karle, E.J.; Büttner, W.: Kariesbefall im Tierversuch nach Verabreichung von Sorbit, Xylit, Lycasin® und Calciumsaccharosephosphat. Dtsch. Zahnärztl. Z. *26:*
1097–1108 (1971).

127 Greenwood, M.; Feigal, R.; Messer, H.: Cariogenic potential of liquid medications
in rats. Caries Res. *18:* 447–449 (1984).

128 Mühlemann, H.R.; Regolati, B.; Marthaler, T.M.: The effect on rat fissure caries of
xylitol and sorbitol. Helv. Odontol. Acta *14:* 48–50 (1970).

129 Van Der Hoeven, J.S.: Cariogenicity of lactitol in program-fed rats. Caries Res. *20:*
441–443 (1986).

130 Havenaar, R.: Effects of intermittent feeding of sugar and sugar substitutes on
experimental caries and the colonization of *Streptococcus mutans* in rats; in Havenaar, R. (ed.): Sugar Substitutes and Dental Caries, pp. 73–79 (Elinkwijk, Utrecht
1984).

131 Karle, E.J.; Gehring, F.: Wirkung der Zuckeraustauschstoffe Fruktose, Sorbit und
Xylit auf Kariesbefall und Plaqueflora der Ratte. Dtsch. Zahnärztl. Z. *30:* 356–363
(1975).

132 Karle, E.J.: Die Kariogenität von Xylit im Tierversuch. Dtsch. Zahnärztl. Z. *32:*
S89–S95 (1977).

133 Karyda-Maniatopoulos, A.-M.: A study of the influence of dietary xylitol on dental
caries and *S. mutans* colonization in the rat; thesis Toronto, p. 225 (1983).

134 Grenby, T.H.; Colley, J.: Dental effects of xylitol compared with other carbohydrates and polyols in the diet of laboratory rats. Arch. Oral Biol. *28:* 745–758
(1983).

135 Hefti, A.: Cariogenicity of topically applied sugar substitutes in rats under restricted
feeding conditions. Caries Res. *14:* 136–140 (1980).

136 Firestone, A.R.; Navia, J.M.: In vivo measurements of sulcal plaque pH in rats after
topical applications of xylitol, sorbitol, glucose, sucrose, and sucrose plus 53 mM
sodium fluoride. J. Dent. Res. *65:* 44–48 (1986).

137 Havenaar, R.; Drost, J.S.; De Stoppelaar, J.D.; Huis in't Veld, J.H.J.; Backer-Dirks,
O.: Potential cariogenicity of Lycasin® 80/55 in comparison to starch, sucrose, xylitol, sorbitol and *L*-sorbose in rats. Caries Res. *18:* 375–384 (1984).

138 Karle, E.J.: Futter- und Wasseraufnahme der Ratte im Registrierapparat. Z. Ver-
suchstierkd. *20:* 95–101 (1978).

139 Havenaar, R.; Boom-Gerats, A.: Eating pattern of Osborne-Mendel rats on a sucrose
diet and a sucrose/xylitol diet. Caries Res. *18:* 536–539 (1984).

140 Slack, G.L.; Millward, E.; Martin, W.J.: The effect of tablets stimulating salivary
flow on the incidence of dental caries. Br. Dent. J. *116:* 105–108 (1964).

141 Møller, I.J.: Sorbitol-containing chewing gum and its significance for caries prevention. Dtsch. Zahnärztl. Z. *32:* suppl. 1, pp. 67–70 (1977).

142 Glass, R.L.: A two-year clinical trial of sorbitol chewing gum. Caries Res. *17:* 365–368 (1983).

143 Richardson, A.S.; Hole, L.W.; McCornbie, F.; Kolthammer, J.: Anticariogenic effect of dicalcium phosphate dihydrate chewing gum: Results after two yars. Can. Dent. Assoc. *38:* 213–218 (1972).

144 Finn, S.B.; Jamison, H.C.: The effect of a dicalcium phosphate chewing gum on caries incidence in children: 30-month results. J. Am. Dent. Assoc. *74:* 987–995 (1967).

145 Banoczy, J.; Hadas, E.; Esztari, I.; Marosi, I.; Fözy, L.; Szanto, S.: Dreijährige Erfahrungen mit Sorbit im klinischen Längsschnitt-Versuch. Kariesprophylaxe *2:* 39–46 (1980).

146 Backer-Dirks, O.: Posteruptive changes in dental enamel. J. Dent. Res. *45:* 503–511 (1966).

147 Arends, J.; Ten Bosch, J.J.: In vivo de- and remineralization of dental enamel; in Leach, S.A. (ed.): Factors Relating to Demineralisation and Remineralisation of the Teeth, pp. 1–11 (IRL Press, Oxford 1986).

148 Carey, C.; Gregory, T.; Rupp, W.; Tatevossian, A.; Vogel, G.L.: The driving forces in human dental plaque fluid for demineralisation and remineralisation of enamel mineral; in Leach, S.A. (ed.): Factors Relating to Demineralisation and Remineralisation of the Teeth, pp. 163–173. (IRL Press, Oxford 1986).

149 Pitts, N.B.: Regression of approximal carious lesions diagnosed from serial standardized bitewing radiographs. Caries Res. *20:* 85–90 (1986).

150 Sreebny, L.M.: Salivary flow and dental caries; in Cariology Today. Int. Congr., Zürich 1983, pp. 56–69 (Karger, Basel 1984).

151 Leach, S.A.; Speechley, J.A.; White, M.J.; Abbott, J.J.: Remineralization in vivo by stimulating salivary flow with Lycasin®: a pilot study; in Leach, S.A. (ed.): Factors Relating to Demineralisation and Remineralisation of the Teeth, pp. 69–79 (IRL Press, Oxford 1986).

152 Bowen, W.H.: The cariostatic effect of calcium glycerophosphate in monkeys. Caries Res. *6:* 43 (1972).

153 Cole, M.F.; Eastoe, J.E.; Curtis, M.A.; Korts, D.C.; Bowen, W.H.: Effects of pyridoxine, phytate and invert sugar on plaque composition and caries activity in the monkey *(Macaca fascicularis).* Caries Res. *14:* 1–15 (1980).

154 Harris, R.; Schamschula, R.G.; Beveridge, J.; Gregory, G.: The cariostatic effect of calcium sucrose phosphate in a group of children aged 5–17 years. IV. Aust. Dent. J. *14:* 42 (1969).

155 Shrestha, B.M.; Mundorff, S.A.; Bibby, B.G.: Preliminary studies on calcium lactate as an anticaries food additive. Caries Res. *16:* 12–17 (1982).

156 Lynch, P.; Schemmel, R.A.; Kabara, J.J.: Anticariogenicity of dietary glycerol monolaurin in rats. Caries Res. *17:* 131–138 (1983).

157 Havenaar, R.: Dental advantages of some bulk sweeteners in laboratory animal trials; in Grenby, T.H. (ed.): Developments in Sweeteners – 3, pp. 189–211 (Elsevier Applied Science, London 1987).

158 Ziesenitz, S.C.: Süssstoffwirkungen auf Mundbakterien und Karies. Dtsch. Zahnärztl. Z. *42:* S113–S123 (1987).

159 Kleinberg, I.: Oral effects of sugars and sweeteners. Int. Dent. J. *35:* 180–189 (1985).

160 Mouton, C.: The efficacy of gum chewing and xylitol to reduce oral glucose clearance time. J. Can. Dent. Assoc. *9:* 655–660 (1983).

161 Edgar, W.M.: The role of saliva in the control of pH changes in human dental plaque. Caries Res. *10:* 241–254 (1976).

162 Abelson, D.C.; Mandel, I.D.: The effect of saliva on plaque pH in vivo. J. Dent. Res. *60:* 1634–1638 (1981).

163 Jensen, M.E.: Effects of chewing sorbitol gum and paraffin on human interproximal plaque pH. Caries Res. *20:* 503–509 (1986).

164 Jensen, M.E.: Interproximal plaque pH: Effects of chewing xylitol-sorbitol gum. J. Dent. Res. *66:* 347, abstr. 1925 (1987).

165 Maiwald, H.-J.; Banoczy, J.; Tietze, W.; Toth, Z.S.; Vegh, A.: Die Beeinflussung des Plaque-pH durch zuckerhaltigen und zuckerfreien Kaugummi. Zahn- Mund- Kieferheilkd. *70:* 598–604 (1982).

166 Hay, D.I.; Schluckebier, S.K.; Moreno, E.C.: Equilibrium dialysis and ultrafiltration studies of calcium and phosphate binding by human salivary protein. Implications from salivary supersaturation with respect to calcium phosphate salts. Calcif. Tissue Int. *34:* 531–538 (1982).

167 Kashket, S.; Yaskell T.; Lopez, L.R.: Prevention of sucrose-induced demineralization of tooth enamel by chewing sorbitol gum. J. Dent. Res. *68:* 460–462 (1989).

168 Leach, S.A.; Agalamanyi, E.A.; Green, R.M.: Remineralisation of the teeth by dietary means; in Leach, S.A.; Edgar, W.M. (eds): Demineralisation and Remineralisation of the Teeth, pp. 51–73 (IRL Press, Oxford 1983).

169 Bowden, G.H.; Milnes, A.R.; Boyar, R.: *Streptococcus mutans* and caries: State of the art 1983; in Cariology Today. Int. Congr., Zürich 1983, pp. 173–181 (Karger, Basel 1984).

170 Minah, G.E.; Lovekin, G.B.; Finney, J.P.: Sucrose-induced ecological response of experimental dental plaques from caries-free and caries-susceptible human volunteers. Infect. Immun. *34:* 662–675 (1981).

171 Scheie, A.A.; Arneberg, P.; Orstavik, D.; Afseth, J.: Microbial composition, pH-depressing capacity and acidogenicity of 3-week smooth surface plaque developed on sucrose-regulated diets in man. Caries Res. *18:* 74–86 (1984).

171 Bibby, B.G.; Fu, J.: Changes in plaque pH in vitro by sweeteners. J. Dent. Res. *64:* 1130–1133 (1985).

173 Assev, S.; Rølla, G.: Sorbitol increases the growth inhibition of xylitol on *S. mutans* OMZ 176. Acta Pathol. Microbiol. Immunol. Scand. *94B:* 231–237 (1986).

174 Sasaki, N.; Topitsoglou, V.; Frostell, G.: Effects of xylitol on the acid production activity from sorbitol by *Streptococcus mutans* and human dental plaque. Swed. Dent. J. *7:* 153–160 (1983).

175 Rölla, G.; Oppermann, R.V.; Waaler, S.M.; Assev, S.: Effect of aqueous solutions of sorbitol-xylitol on plaque metabolism and on growth of *Streptococcus mutans.* Scand. J. Dent. Res. *89:* 247–250 (1981).

176 Lohmann, D.; Gehring, F.; Bär, A.: Effect of xylitol on fermentation of sorbitol by *S. mutans* (abstract). J. Dent. Res. *59:* 1867 (1980).

177 Kandelman, D.; Gagnon, G.: Effect on dental caries of xylitol chewing gum: Two-year results. J. Dent. Res. *67:* 172, abstr. 472 (1988).

178 Shyu, K.-W.; Hsu, M.-Y.: The cariogenicity of xylitol, mannitol, sorbitol and sucrose. Proc. Natl. Sci. Counc. ROC *4:* 21–26 (1980).

179 Kleiner, F.W.; Kinkel, H.-J.: Ernährungsfaktoren bei Zahn- und Knochenbildung. VIII. Dtsch. Zahnärztl. Z. *15:* 664–669 (1960).
180 Grenby, T.H.: Dental effects of Lycasin® in the diet of laboratory rats. Caries Res. *22:* 288–296 (1988).
181 Firestone, A.R.; Schmid, R.; Mühlemann, H.R.: The effects of topical applications of sugar substitutes on the incidence of caries and bacterial agglomerate formation in rats. Caries Res. *14:* 324–332 (1980).
182 Gey, F.; Kinkel, H.T.: Topical application of xylitol and sucrose substitutes after restricted cariogenic meals. J. Dent. Res. *57:* 111, abstr. 147 (1978).
183 Lout, R.K.; Messer, L.B.; Soberay, A.; Kajander, K.; Rudney, J.: Cariogenicity of frequent aspartame and sorbitol rinsing in laboratory rats. Caries Res. *22:* 237–241 (1988).
184 Scheinin, A.; Mäkinen K.K.; Tamisalo, E.; Rekola, M.: Turku sugar studies. XVIII. Incidence of dental caries in relation to 1-year consumption of xylitol chewing gum. Acta Odont. Scand. *33:* 269–278 (1975).

Dowen Birkhed, DDS, Odont. Dr., Department of Cariology,
University of Göteborg, PO Box 33070, S–400 33 Göteborg (Sweden)

Simopoulos AP (ed): Impacts on Nutrition and Health.
World Rev Nutr Diet. Basel, Karger, 1991, vol 65, pp 38–71

Moderate Alcohol Use and Coronary Heart Disease: A U-Shaped Curve?

Jan Veenstra[1]

TNO-CIVO Toxicology and Nutrition Institute, Department of Nutrition,
Zeist, The Netherlands

Contents

[1] Prof Dr. Ir. R.J.J. Hermus, Dr. Ir. G. Schaafsma, Dr. Th. Ockhuizen, who are all involved in alcohol research in our institute, and D.G. van der Heÿ are gratefully acknowledged for their support in writing the manuscript.

Introduction

About 40–50% of total mortality in the affluent society is caused by cardiovascular disease (CVD). Most of the CVD death cases can be attributed to coronary heart disease (CHD). In the past decades evidence has been found that life-style factors influence the risk of CHD. Besides smoking, lack of physical exercise, stress, and a surplus of dietary cholesterol, saturated fatty acids, salt and energy contribute to a higher risk of CHD.

Excessive alcohol use is another CHD risk factor. In contrast, in the past decade, moderate alcohol use has frequently been claimed to reduce this risk. The association between alcohol consumption and CHD risk or between alcohol consumption and total mortality has often been reported to be U-shaped, i.e. moderate drinkers would be at lower risk than both teetotallers and heavy drinkers.

This paper aims at critically reviewing the literature on this subject and finding an answer to the question whether the association between CHD and alcohol use is U-shaped indeed. On the basis of epidemiological and experimental studies those mechanisms are discussed that could explain such a U-shaped curve.

Epidemiological Research on Alcohol and CHD

In many epidemiological studies an inverse correlation between moderate alcohol use and CHD incidence has been found. These studies can be classified into ecological studies, case-control studies and cohort studies.

Ecological Studies
A number of ecological studies have investigated the relation between average alcohol consumption and CHD prevalence in various countries. In 1969, Brummer [1] compared alcohol consumption and CHD mortality data of 20 Western countries. An inverse association between alcohol consumption and CHD mortality was observed for both men and women in three different age categories. St. Leger et al. [2], in a comparable study, investigated CHD mortality among men and women aged 55–64 in 18 countries. In this study, alcohol was classified into wine, beer and spirits. A clear inverse relation between average total alcohol consumption and CHD mortality was found. Besides, St. Leger et al. observed that the effect of alcohol was not attributable to differences in known risk factors of CHD

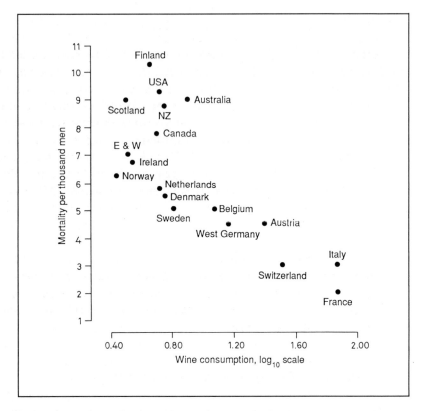

Fig. 1. Relationship between CHD mortality rate in men aged 55–64 and wine consumption [2].

such as smoking, cholesterol intake, fat intake or total energy intake. Wine appeared to be the predominant form of alcohol responsible for the favourable effect of alcohol consumption (fig. 1).

Comparable results have been reported by LaPorte et al. [3], Hegsted and Ausman [4], and Schmidt and Popham [5]. Schmidt and Popham also reported significant negative correlations between the consumption of total alcohol, wine and spirits and CHD mortality in the 50 states of the USA. LaPorte et al. [3] have also paid attention to trends in alcohol use and CHD incidence rates. The strongest relation they found applied for beer. Figure 2 presents the relation between average beer consumption (1945–1975) and CHD mortality (1950–1975) in the USA. Taking into

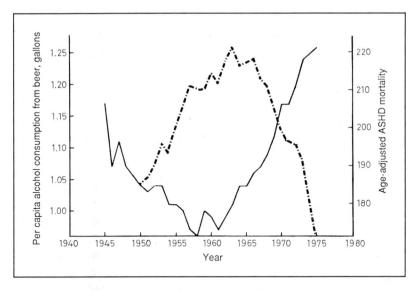

Fig. 2. Relationship of changes in adult per capita intake of alcohol beer (1945–1975) to changes in total United States age-adjusted heart disease death rates (1950–1975). ▬·▬ = CHD death rate; ▬▬▬ = beer consumption [3].

account a 5-year lag period, the correlation coefficient between beer consumption and CHD mortality was −0.943. The predictive value of beer consumption appeared to be even higher than that of fat consumption and smoking. A similar pattern was found for total alcohol consumption.

Ecological studies are no real proof of a favourable effect of alcohol consumption on CHD development. Results just indicate a relationship on a population level, and differences between countries with regard to culture and living and working conditions are not taken into account. A second drawback of these studies is that alcohol consumption data are derived from alcohol sales data, uncorrected for sales to visitors from abroad.

Finally, the hypothetical U-shaped curve poses an insurmountable problem for ecological studies since the use of sales statistics does not differentiate between nondrinkers, moderate drinkers and heavy drinkers.

In spite of these objections, the fact that the CHD mortality rate for Frenchmen aged 55–64 is so much (almost 3-fold) lower than for their Dutch contemporaries is most intriguing and suggests the need for further research.

Case-Control Studies

In many case-control studies alcohol consumption among CHD cases has been compared with that among controls [6–13]. The results of these studies fairly consistently point at an inverse relation between moderate alcohol consumption and CHD incidence for both men and women. Only Kaufman et al. [13] found no effect of moderate alcohol consumption.

Petitti et al. [9] found among women the relative risk (RR) of acute myocardial infarction for nondrinkers versus drinkers to be 3.1 (95% CI (confidence interval) 1.6–6.0). These results were confirmed by Stason et al. [6] for both men and women. In another study among women, Rosenberg et al. [11] arrived at similar conclusions; they found significantly lower RRs among drinkers for wine, beer and spirits separately (0.5, 0.8, 0.9, respectively).

The studies mentioned above have not differentiated for consumption level. Hennekens et al. [7], however, classified their study population into three categories, with an average daily consumption of 0, 0–3½ and > 3½ glasses, respectively). The relative risk was found to be significantly lower for moderate drinkers than for nondrinkers (RR = 0.4), but the difference between the highest consumption category and the nondrinkers was not significant (RR = 0.7). In contrast, Klatsky et al. [8] found the relative risk to decrease with increasing consumption level (0.4, 0.7 and 1.0 for categories with a daily consumption level of > 5, 3–5 and < 3 glasses, respectively).

As for ecological studies, some critical comments could be made on case-control studies. First, many case-control studies have been conducted in a hospital, so that CHD patients dying before arrival at the hospital have been left aside. However, the results of two studies in which the CHD cases who had died before admission were included [7, 9] did not diverge from other results.

Second, the group defined as 'nondrinkers at the time of investigation' may comprise former alcoholics who have recently stopped drinking alongside people who have never drunk. Since the group of nondrinkers is usually the reference group (RR = 1.0) this classification bias can yield erroneous results. Klatsky et al. [8], therefore, defined nondrinkers as people who had not drunk any alcohol in the past year at least, and the control group of Rosenberg et al. [11] comprised exclusively lifelong teetotallers. In both studies an inverse relationship between moderate alcohol consumption and CHD incidence could still be found.

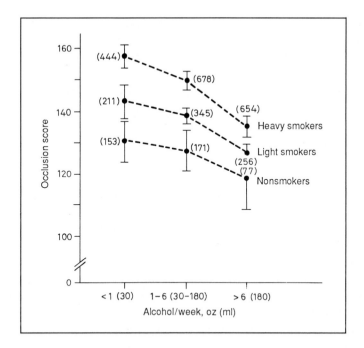

Fig. 3. Interrelationships between the extent of coronary occlusion, alcohol intake and smoking. Number of patients in parentheses. Vertical bars = SEM [14].

Third, the category of moderate drinkers could be characterized by a life-style leading to a reduced risk of CHD, regardless of drinking pattern.

In some studies of CHD cases the extent of occlusion of coronary arteries has been established by arteriography [14–17]. Barboriak et al. [14] have studied the effects of smoking and of alcohol consumption on coronary artery occlusion in a group of 2,989 men. Figure 3 summarizes the results of that study. Smoking was found to have a dose-dependent occlusive effect, whereas the effect of alcohol was associated with lower occlusion scores in nonsmokers, light smokers as well as heavy smokers. Gruchow et al. [16] have investigated, within the same study framework, the effect of alcohol consumption pattern by classifying the subjects into nondrinkers, occasional drinkers, regular drinkers adhering to a more or less fixed dose, and regular drinkers varying the amounts consumed. Regular users of moderate doses of alcohol were found to be at significantly lower risk of occlusion of coronary arteries. Irregular drinkers were at higher risk irrespective of dose.

Fried et al. [18] have studied in a group of 31 men with coronary arteries of normal diameter the effects of smoking and of alcohol consumption on the diameter of three main coronary arteries. Smoking and alcohol use appeared to affect these diameters highly singificantly and independently. Smoking was found to have a vasoconstrictive effect, whereas alcohol consumption promoted vasodilatation.

Cohort Studies

In cohort studies, also called prospective studies or longitudinal studies, large study populations are classified into categories varying in alcohol consumption level. After a number of years the association between alcohol consumption and CHD incidence is studied. In the past few years the effect of moderate drinking on CHD incidence has been investigated in many cohorts all over the world [19–45]. A reduced risk of CHD has been found among moderate drinkers in Framingham, Mass. [19, 39, 40], Chicago [25], San Francisco [26, 27], western Australia [28], Yugoslavia [29], eastern Finland [30], Puerto Rico [31], Albany, N.Y. [32], London [33] and Japan [34, 35].

In two studies – one in Ireland [36], another in California [37] – no effects of alcohol use were found. A recent study in Finland showed, in contrast to all other studies, a positive association between consumption of alcohol, in particular consumption of spirits, and CHD incidence [38].

It is from cohort studies in particular that the U-shaped curve has arisen. In 1980, Dyer et al. [25], who had followed 1,899 employees of the Western Electric Company from 1957 to 1974, were the first to suggest the U-shaped curve. They found CHD incidence to decrease with increasing alcohol consumption up to a daily dose of 5 glasses and to increase at higher dosages. However these results lost their significance after correction for smoking habits, serum cholesterol level and blood pressure. In 1981 the U-shaped curve was confirmed by Klatsky et al. [26], who had followed 8,060 Californian men and women for 10 years, and by Marmot et al. [33] in a comparable study among 1,422 male civil servants in London (fig. 4).

In the study of Marmot et al. the decreasing left-hand part of the U-shaped curve was attributed primarily to a decrease in CVD mortality rate with increasing alcohol consumption, and the increasing right-hand part to an increase in mortality unrelated to CVD at an average daily

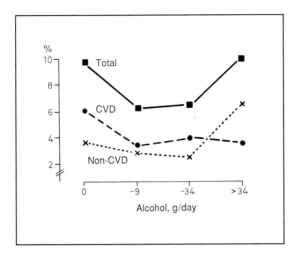

Fig. 4. Relationship between 10-year mortality (CVD- and non-CVD-related) and daily alcohol consumption [33].

alcohol dose above 34 g. In 1986, Friedman and Kimball [39] found support for a U-shaped association between alcohol consumption and CHD incidence in their study among 5,209 men and women in Framingham during a 24-year follow-up period. The decreased CHD incidence among moderate drinkers as compared to nondrinkers has been confirmed in various other studies (see above).

A serious drawback of many of these studies is that the category of nondrinkers considered in these studies may comprise former heavy drinkers as well as people who have given up alcohol on medical advice based, for example, on a heart condition. This possible bias has recently been studied by Shaper et al. [41] in a cohort of 7,735 men living in 24 different towns in England, Scotland and Wales. They found a U-shaped relationship between alcohol consumption and total mortality and an inverse relationship between alcohol consumption and CVD mortality, in fair correspondence with the results of Marmot et al. (fig. 4). At the start of the follow-up study, when the average age of the subjects was 50 years, 24.2% of the subjects had a heart condition. The associations between alcohol and total mortality and between alcohol and CVD mortality were studied for both subcohorts separately (men suffering from and men free from heart disorders). In the category initially free from heart disorders a U-shaped or inverse relationship could no longer be found. Shaper et al. concluded that the U-shaped curve could largely be explained from the fact that people suffering from CVD disorders tend to reduce or even give up alcohol consumption so that the curvature cannot be attributed to any favourable effects of moderate alcohol use. The *Lancet* paper of Shaper et al. [41] has evoked a lively discussion in that journal as to whether moderate alcohol use protects against CHD [42–44].

In the Honolulu Heart Study [23], in which the nondrinkers were classified into lifetime teetotallers and former drinkers, a higher CHD incidence as compared to drinkers was found for both categories. This finding has been supported by the results of a case-control study among 513 cases and 918 controls [11] and other studies [27, 34, 35]. In the Honolulu Heart Study [23] and in a study by Klatsky et al. [27] no significant differences in CHD risk were found between lifetime teetotallers and former drinkers. Finally, Stampfer et al. [45], in a cohort of as many as 87,526 nurses, has recently searched into any changes in drinking habits over the past 10 years. Subjects who had given up drinking on medical advice could be excluded from the study this way. The CHD risk for the nondrinkers group were found to be up to 2½ times as high as for the drinkers categories.

The results of the various studies are less consistent for the right-hand part of the U-shaped curve, i.e. the higher CHD risk for excessive drinkers. Some studies, however, work with relatively low upper limits. In the study of Marmot et al. [33], for example, all people with a daily alcohol consumption over 34 g have been assigned to one and the same category (fig. 4), although adverse effects of alcohol use on CHD may apply for far higher levels.

In most cohort studies alcoholic beverages are not categorized. However, there are marked (culturally based) differences in popularity of particular beverages, which could be reflected by the results of the various studies.

Summary

In most epidemiological studies an inverse relationship between moderate alcohol use and CHD incidence has been found. In some studies excessive alcohol use has been found to increase CHD risk, which could imply a U-shaped, or J-shaped, relationship. All three types of study – ecological, case-control and cohort studies – are subject to criticism. The strongest objection against these types of research could be that the association between alcohol consumption and CHD found may well be attributable to factors other than alcohol, such as differences in personality, life-style or nutrition, or a combination of these. If so, these unknown factors must increase CHD risk for nondrinkers in populations as diverse as Japanese in Japan, Japanese in Hawaii, people in various regions of the USA, Puerto Ricans, Yugoslavians, London civil servants, and inhabitants of Busselton, Australia. Moreover, these factors must be most dominant in countries with the lowest alcohol consumption. Of course, such factors or such a complex of factors could exist. However, a preventive effect of moderate alcohol use on CHD far more simply explains the effects observed.

The question how moderate alcohol use can influence CHD risk is discussed below.

Epidemiological Research into CHD Risk Factors

Several factors have been found to influence CHD risk. In search of explanations for the favourable effect of moderate alcohol use on CHD risk many epidemiologists have studied the relationships between alcohol use and these risk factors.

Blood Pressure

The popularity of blood pressure measurements in population research is reflected by the large number of epidemiological studies on the relationship between alcohol use and blood pressure. As early as 1915, Camille Lian [46] reported an elevated blood pressure as a result of excessive alcohol use. Many epidemiological studies have fairly consistently confirmed the hypertensive effect of excessive alcohol use [47–55], even after correction for other CHD risk factors such as smoking, obesity, excessive salt intake and high serum cholesterol level.

There is much less consensus as to the question of the level at which alcohol consumption has a hypertensive effect. Some studies have found a continuous increase, from no alcohol use to heavy use [47, 48, 58, 59]. Some other studies have established a threshold above which alcohol use was found to be positively associated with blood pressure. In still other studies [51, 52, 60] a J-shaped relationship between alcohol use and blood pressure was found, in particular for women (fig. 5).

So, it is hard to tell whether or to what extent moderate alcohol use contributes to hypertension incidence. Hypertension increases CHD risk, but moderate alcohol use is certainly not positively related to CHD incidence. Hypertension also increases the risk of cerebral haemorrhage, which appears to be positively related to excessive alcohol use [61–63].

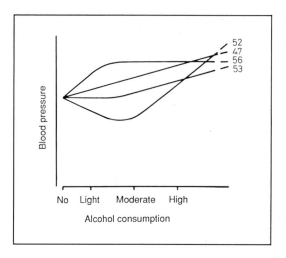

Fig. 5. Relationship between alcohol consumption and blood pressure in different studies [47, 52, 53, 56, 57].

Cholesterol Metabolism

Cholesterol is a well-known CHD risk factor. An essential element in the body's defence against cholesterol accumulation in tissues – where cholesterol can damage vascular wall – is 'reverse cholesterol transport', i.e., transport from the tissues to the liver, where cholesterol is converted into bile acids and excreted via the bile. The lipoprotein that probably plays an important role in this reverse cholesterol transport is high-density lipoprotein (HDL). HDL consists of proteins for about 50%, among which apolipoproteins A_1 and A_2 (Apo-A_1 and Apo-A_2) are predominant. These proteins are essential not only as an envelope for lipids to be transported but also for particle recognition.

Epidemiological studies [64–71] have established that a high blood HDL-cholesterol (HDL-C) level decreases CVD risk. Apo-A_1 and Apo-A_2 concentrations may be even better indicators of CVD risk. A great deal of epidemiological studies [72–95] all over the world have consistently proved a positive association between alcohol consumption and blood HDL-C level. When the research populations were classified according to gender and type of alcoholic beverage consumed (fig. 6), as in the Tromsø Heart Study [77], the correlations in all categories were significantly positive. Even low alcohol doses increased HDL-C levels.

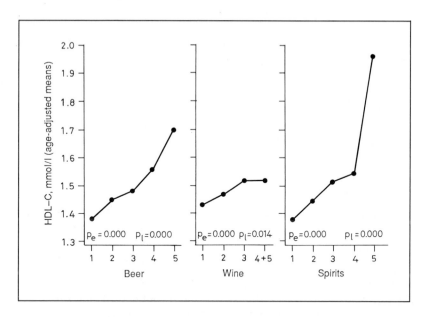

Fig. 6. Relationship between HDL-C (●——●) and alcohol consumption [77]. p_e = p value for test of equal group means; p_l = p value for test of linear trend.

One could wonder whether this apparently linear relationship between alcohol consumption and blood HDL-C level can explain a favourable effect of alcohol use on CHD incidence. Initially it seemed so in view of the increase of the HDL-C level induced by alcohol consumption. Later doubts about the protective effect of alcohol along the HDL-C pathway are based on the fact that HDL-C consists of two subfractions, HDL_2-C and HDL_3-C. In epidemiological studies HDL_2-C has been associated with CHD risk, but HDL_3-C far less so [96]. The increase of the HDL-C induced by moderate alcohol use, however, has been attributed predominantly to the HDL_3-C fraction [96] whereas elevated values for HDL_2-C – the subfraction most related to CHD risk – have been found particularly in alcoholics. Alcoholics, however, run highly increased health risks along other pathways and hence draw little benefit from an increased HDL_2-C level. Recently, however, Miller et al. [97], in the first large-scale epidemiological study (4,860 men) on the effects of alcohol on HDL-C subfraction levels, found comparable positive associations between alcohol consumption and both HDL_2-C and HDL_3-C.

Few epidemiologists studying the effects of moderate alcohol use have taken the apoproteins Apo-A_1 and Apo-A_2 into consideration. Phillips et al. [98] have found a positive association between alcohol use and Apo-A_1 level in a group of 289 Californian men and women, but have not measured Apo-A_2. Haffner et al. [99] (77 men) and Williams et al. [95] (50 men and women) have found positive correlations for both Apo-A_1 and Apo-A_2. In these two studies alcohol use was found to correlate positively with HDL_3-C level, but not with HDL_2-C level.

Haemostasis

Besides impairment of vascular walls, haemostasis plays an important part in the occurrence of a myocardial or cerebral infarction. Haemostasis is the balance between clot formation, in which blood platelets are involved, and fibrinolysis, the dissolution of such clots. In a study into the causes of occlusion of coronary arteries in cases of myocardial infarction, in most cases the artery was found to be blocked by a clot primarily consisting of thrombocytes [100]. In normal physiological conditions the formation of thrombocyte clots, called platelet aggregation, is continually inhibited by prostacyclin, a substance formed by endothelial cells covering the blood vessels. The platelets themselves produce thromboxane, which stimulates platelet aggregation. Most probably, platelets constantly aggregate to some extent, depending on the balance of thromboxane and prostacycline production. Besides, several fibrinolytic factors play a part in continually dissolving newly formed clots.

Recently a large-scale epidemiological study proved that influencing the thromboxane/prostacyclin balance by a dose of 350 mg aspirin every other day favourably affects myocardial infarction risk [101]. A lowered fibrinolytic activity has been found in infarct patients [102–106]. Good results have been achieved in stimulating fibrinolytic activity immediately upon occurrence of the infarct and thus making the clot blocking the blood vessel redissolve [107]. Of course, if alcohol influences this complex and delicate haemostatic balance this could explain the favourable effect of alcohol consumption on CHD risk.

In epidemiological studies on the physiological consequences of moderate alcohol use hardly any research effort has been devoted to the platelet aggregation process. Epidemiological research in this field is primarily hampered by analytical problems. Most analytical methods for the measurement of thrombocyte function are complicated and time-consuming, and analyses must be carried out soon (within 1 h) after blood sampling, which makes analyses of this kind hard to use in large-scale population studies. That is why only one research team has included this variable in their study. Maede et al. [108] have investigated the association between alcohol consumption and platelet aggregation in a population of 685 British men and 273 British women (Northwick Park Heart Study). They found an inverse relationship for both adenosine diphosphate (ADP)-induced and adrenaline-induced platelet aggregation.

Some new analytical methods for determining platelet function are easier to use in large study populations and are likely to be used in future epidemiological alcohol studies, e.g. the platelet factor β-thromboglobulin and platelet factor 4 (PF-4), which are indicators of in vivo platelet aggregation. To date, however, investigations into the association between alcohol use and platelet function are almost exclusively confined to experimental research.

Maede et al. [109] have also investigated the effect of alcohol on fibrinolysis in men and women of the Northwick Park Heart Study population. They found moderate alcohol use to be associated with a decreased plasma fibrinogen level and an increased fibrinolytic activity.

Summary

In epidemiological research on the association between alcohol use and CHD risk indicators a number of possible explanations of the beneficial effect of moderate alcohol use on CHD incidence have been studied. Excessive alcohol use has been found to elevate blood pressure. The effect of moderate alcohol use on blood pressure is still uncertain. Alcohol use affects cholesterol metabolism. Moderate alcohol use appears to be associated with an increased HDL-C level. Initially this increase was assumed to (partly) explain the favourable effects of moderate alcohol use. Later, moderate alcohol use has been found to be associated primarily with an increase of the HDL_3-C fraction, whereas it is the other fraction, HDL_2-C, that is claimed to have a beneficial effect on CHD risk. However, alcohol consumption has recently been proved to be positively associated with both HDL_2-C and HDL_3-C. In addition, alcohol can affect cholesterol metabolism favourably by increasing the levels of Apo-A_1 and Apo-A_2 apolipoproteins.

Alcohol might also protect against CHD by influencing haemostasis. Just one research group has paid attention to the effects of alcohol on platelet aggregation and found an inverse relationship between alcohol use and platelet aggregation rate.

In one epidemiological study, in which fibrinolysis was among the subjects of investigation, evidence has been produced that moderate alcohol use is associated with an increase of fibrinolytic activity, thereby promoting the efficient removal of clots from the circulation.

Experimental Research on CHD Risk Factors

An association between alcohol use and CHD risk has been demonstrated in many epidemiological studies. Other epidemiological work suggests that alcohol consumption influences several CHD risk factors. However, in these observational studies it is difficult to assess the possible causal nature of the associations seen.

Experimental research enables the establishment of the direct effect of a particular treatment on variables such as blood pressure, cholesterol metabolism indices and haemostasis. However, experimental studies have their limitations as well. Such experiments are usually confined to a period of a few weeks, and long-term effects cannot be pronounced upon. In contrast, in epidemiological research effects and between-group differences can be surveyed over many years or even during a lifetime. Further, experimental studies are conducted in selected groups of limited size. Experimental alcohol studies are often confined to only one beverage type and one or two dosages. In experimental research, therefore, the study design should be chosen such that relevant conclusions on the effects of moderate alcohol use can be given in spite of the limitations mentioned.

Blood Pressure

In experimental research the effect of alcohol on blood pressure has been studied for normotensive subjects, hypertensive subjects as well as CHD patients. Potter et al. [110] have studied the effect of a single alcohol dose on the blood pressure of 16 young male students. Blood pressure was measured over a 5-hour period after the ingestion of either 600 ml nonalcoholic beer or 600 ml nonalcoholic beer spiked with alcohol (0.75 g/kg body weight). All volunteers were subjected to both treatments in a crossover design. The period between both treatments was at least 1 week. The blood pressure course roughly paralleled the blood alcohol level: after a rapid increase by ca. 7 mm Hg within 1 h blood pressure gradually decreased. Similar acute effects have been observed by Ireland et al. [111, 112]. Studies of this design have the drawback that the two treatments are not isocaloric: the caloric value of the alcohol is not compensated for in the control treatment. In a study by Stott et al. [113] this energy effect has been taken into account. In their study, the design of which was comparable to that of Potter et al. [110] for the rest, an isocaloric amount of glucose was added to the nonalcoholic drink. A slight increase of blood pressure was observed 1 h after alcohol ingestion, followed by a decrease. However, the picture was similar for the glucose treatment. Stott et al. [113] concluded that the increase of blood pressure after the ingestion of a single moderate dose of alcohol does not differ from the decrease after the ingestion of an isocaloric amount of glucose.

An increase in plasma adrenaline and noradrenaline levels after alcohol ingestion found in some studies [112, 114–116] have been connected with a rise in blood pressure. However, these studies have not allowed for the caloric value of alcohol, in spite of indications that energy intake alone can increase plasma catecholamine level [117]. Further, rapid ingestion of alcohol in experimental conditions can evoke a specific stress response and feelings of discomfort [118]. Stott et al. [113], who have allowed for these aspects as far as possible, have not found effects of alcohol consumption on plasma catecholamine level.

In various investigations the effects of alcohol consumption on the blood pressure of hypertensive subjects have been studied [119–121]. Puddy et al. [119], in a study among 44 hypertensives accustomed to the daily consumption of at least 3 glasses of alcoholic beverage (6–7 glasses on the average), investigated the effect of the consumption of low-alcohol beer (0.9% v/v alcohol) versus regular beer (5% v/v alcohol). After a 6-week period in which they consumed regular beer in amounts equivalent to the alcohol dose they were accustomed to they switched over to low-alcohol beer for another 6-week period. Their blood pressure was found to be significantly higher in the period of regular beer consumption. Similar results among hypertensives have been found by Potter and Beevers [120] and Malhotra et al. [121], albeit over shorter periods (4 and 5 days respectively). In the study of Puddy et al. [119] not only blood pressure but also body weight was significantly higher in the period of regular beer consumption. This body weight increase has undoubtedly strengthened the effect of alcohol on blood pressure. To date no studies among hypertensives have been conducted in which the effect of alcohol energy versus nonalcohol energy has been investigated.

Kelbaek et al. [122, 123] have recently studied the effect of a single alcohol dose (0.9 g/kg body weight) on the heart function of 20 male CHD and cardiopathy patients. Ten controls with a similar clinical picture received an equal amount of an isocaloric nonalcoholic drink. A slight but significant decrease (6%) of the systemic arterial blood pressure was found after alcohol ingestion. Alcohol was found to have no effect on the central venous pressure, on pulmonary artery pressure, on cardiac output, on stroke volume or on global peripheral resistance. Kelbaek et al. concluded that ingestion of a moderate dose of alcohol by CHD patients is unlikely to evoke disease symptoms.

Cholesterol Metabolism

Experimental studies into the effect of alcohol use on cholesterol metabolism can be classified in various ways, for example according to experimental period, alcohol dose, beverage type or variables measured. Besides, in some studies alcoholics have been included.

In many studies a promotive effect of alcohol on HDL or HDL-C level has been found within some weeks after alcohol ingestion [124–133]. Only two studies have not found any effect [134, 135]. However, it should be noted that the experimental period was rather short in one of these studies [134] and that the alcohol dose was very low in the other one [135]. Moore et al. [135] did find an increased Apo-A_1 level after a daily consumption of 1 glass of beer for 8 weeks. Table 1 surveys the doses and beverage types applied in the studies mentioned and the lenght of the experimental periods.

The HDL-C fractions HDL_2-C and HDL_3-C have been determined separately in six studies [126, 128–130, 132, 135]. The results of these studies are conflicting. Haskell et al. [126] and Pikaar et al. [130] have found an increase of HDL_3-C, but not of HDL_2-C. Burr et al. [128] and

Table 1. Survey of studies into the effects of some weeks of alcohol use on HDL or HDL-C level

Alcohol dose g/day	Type of beverage	Duration of study weeks	Reference
28	beer	3	124
39	white wine	6	125
31 (average)	optional	6	126
31	red wine	5	127
18.4 (average)	optional	4	128
24	beer	6	129
23 or 46	red wine	5	130
75	alcohol or beer	5	131
75	red wine	5	132
90	dilute alcohol	4	133
34 or 53	vodka	2	134
12.6	beer	8	135

Contaldo et al. [132], however, have reported that the HDL-C rise found in their studies could be attributed primarily to an increase of HDL_2-C level. Masarei et al. [129] have found significant increases for both HDL_2-C and HDL_3-C. Moore et al. [135] have not found an effect of alcohol on HDL-C, nor on any of its fractions.

Apo-A_1 levels have been determined in just three of the above papers [127, 129, 135] and Apo-A_2 in just one of these [129]. Alcohol has consistently been found to increase Apo-A_1 levels, and in the study of Masarei et al. [129] Apo-A_2 levels were found to be significantly higher after beer consumption for 6 weeks. Camargo et al. [136] have studied the effect of alcohol (3 weeks, 37.8 ml on the average) on apolipoproteins in 24 healthy volunteers and found similar results for both Apo-A_1 and Apo-A_2.

Increased HDL-C levels are frequently found in alcoholics. In some studies the course of the HDL levels over a period of abstention has been studied. Välimäki et al. [137] have studied the changes in blood lipid levels in 12 alcoholics who had presented themselves for therapy in an alcohol rehabilitation centre at Helsinki. All of them were still under the influence of alcohol at the start of the study. As soon as 2 days after the start of abstention a significant decrease was found for levels of HDL_2 (16%), HDL_2-C (30%) and HDL_3-C (14%). HDL_2 and HDL_2-C levels continued to decrease in the next days to a total decrease of 38 and 47% respectively. The effects observed in the HDL_2 fraction were much stronger than those for HDL_3, which made the authors conclude that changes in HDL in chronic alcoholics are primarily explained by changes in HDL_2. The rapid decline of HDL-C levels found leads to the conclusion that increased HDL-C levels are maintained only as long as alcohol is consumed on a regular basis and return to normal levels upon abstention. The decrease of HDL levels in alcoholics upon abstention has been confirmed by other studies [138–143]. The HDL_2 and HDL_3 fractions have only been studied separately in a study by Taskinen et al. [143], who belonged to the same research group as Välimäki et al. [137]. Changes upon abstention were found to apply primarily to the HDL_2 fraction in this study too.

The observed short-term effects in alcoholics during abstention was the reason for another study by Välimäki et al. [144] in which the effects of moderate (30 g/day) and heavy alcohol consumption (60 g/day) were compared. The consumption levels differed in their effect on the HDL fractions. The high level increased HDL_2 levels within 2 days and gradually increased HDL_3 levels later on, whereas the lower level affected HDL_3 levels only.

In all studies mentioned above, blood lipid levels have been determined in the fasting state, usually after an overnight fast. Recently some
groups have studied the acute effects of alcohol on blood lipid levels in the
postprandial state. Goldberg et al. [145] and Franceschini et al. [146],
using a comparable experimental design, have studied the effects of a single dose of 40 g alcohol. The alcohol (120 ml whisky) was drunk at 09.00 h
after a 14-hour fast. In the study of Franceschini et al., 100 g mayonnaise
and 25 g bread were combined with the whisky. Blood lipid levels were
measured 4, 6, 8, 10 and 12 h after breakfast. Both studies departed from
the assumption that the alcohol had been fully metabolized after 4 h. Goldberg et al. found a significant increase of HDL-C level after alcohol consumption. Moreover, the activity of hepatic lipase, an enzyme essential to
reverse cholesterol transport, was found to have decreased by 67%. Franceschini et al. found a decrease of HDL-C level after consumption of alcohol, mayonnaise and bread relative to the treatment without alcohol.

Recently in our Department of Nutrition, studies have been performed on the effects of moderate alcohol use in the postprandial phase,
1 h after alcohol ingestion when the blood alcohol concentration is
assumed to peak. To date no studies seem to have considered the possibility that the contended favourable effect of moderate alcohol use on cholesterol metabolism is effective when the alcohol is still in the circulation. In
our studies the effects of a moderate alcohol dose have been investigated in
a situation approximating reality as far as possible. In one of these studies
[manuscript in press in Alcohol Alcoholism], each of 8 men aged 20–30
and 8 men aged 45–55 combined alcohol consumption with a dinner early
in the evening. Half an hour before dinner they drunk 1 glass of port, and
during dinner 2 glasses of red wine. For comparison, they drank similar
amounts of mineral water instead of alcohol on another day. One hour
after dinner, we found higher HDL-C levels for the alcohol treatment than
for the mineral water treatment. The HDL-C-promoting effect was more
prominent in the middle-aged men and was most evident for the HDL$_2$-C
fraction.

Haemostasis

In experimental research attention has also been paid to effects of
alcohol on haemostasis. Research on platelet function is characterized by
broad variation in methodology. The most commonly used parameter is
platelet aggregation. In a platelet suspension in plasma aggregation is
induced by adding collagen or another catalyst. Collagen induces platelet

aggregation also under physiological conditions, when tissue damage leads to haemorrhage. Besides, aggregation can be induced by many other stimuli. A serious drawback of determinations of this type is that the results of in vitro measurements of platelet function are not necessarily applicable to the in vivo situation. First, stimulation of platelet aggregation in vitro asks for stimulus levels far above physiological concentrations. Second, the platelet-rich plasma suspension contains no cells but platelets, whereas aggregation in vivo is a combined action of various types of blood cells and endothelial cells of the vascular wall, in which a regulatory role is played by the various mediators produced by these cells. Third, the risk of an infarct is determined by the spontaneous tendency towards aggregation of the platelets in vivo, which can be started off by a shift in haemostatic balance. No reliable conclusions with regard to this process can be drawn from in vitro determinations of platelet aggregation.

Bleeding time is the time after which a wound (puncture or incision) stops bleeding. The drawbacks of platelet aggregation measurements mentioned above do not apply to this parameter. However, measurement of bleeding time is imprecise and hard to standardize.

Finally, statements as to the tendency towards aggregation can also be given on the basis of the activity of the aggregation promoter thromboxane and of the aggregation inhibitor prostacyclin.

Table 2 summarizes studies into the effects of alcohol consumption by healthy volunteers on platelet function. From this table it can be concluded that, in spite of the multiplicity of studies in this area, there is still lack of clarity as to the effects of alcohol on platelet function. In some studies considerable amounts of alcohol were consumed. Hillbom et al. [156, 157] have found in two studies an increase of the tendency towards aggregation after a single alcohol dose of 1.5 g/kg body weight. In a subsequent study of similar design [158] they have not found an effect after ingestion of 1.1 g/kg body weight. In accordance with Hillbom et al., Kangasaho et al. [149] have reported an increase of ADP-induced thromboxane production, but they have found lower thromboxane and prostacyclin concentrations in plasma after ingestion of a high dose of alcohol. Provided stimulation during blood sampling is avoided, plasma analysis can produce an indication of in vivo concentrations of these mediators. Landolfi et al. [153] have observed an increase of plasma prostacyclin level after ingestion of a moderate dose of alcohol (32 g). An increased prostacyclin production by endothelial cells [160] and by leucocytes [161] has also been demonstrated in vitro. Elmér et al. [152] have found an extended bleeding time in connection with a lowered aggregation tendency after ingestion of a single dose of 0.64 g alcohol/kg body weight.

The study of Pikaar et al. [130] is the only one we know of in which the effect of alcohol consumption has been studied over a longer period (5 weeks). In this study, carried out in our Department, a decrease in platelet aggregation was found at a time at which no alcohol was present in the circulation. In a sequel to this study no effects were observed within a 4-day period of moderate alcohol consumption, which could indicate that the acute effects observed result in a permanent decrease of aggregation tendency on the long run. This hypothesis is supported by the results of the epidemiological study of Meade et al. [108] who have found an inverse relation between alcohol and platelet aggregation tendency. So far, virtually all research has focused on acute effects of – usually excessive – alcohol doses. More research is needed to arrive at definite conclusions as to the effect of moderate alcohol use on platelet function, particularly to the effect on the longer run.

Table 2. Survey of studies into the effects of alcohol use on platelet function

Ref.	Year of investigation	Number of volunteers	Alcohol dose, g	Term	Parameter	Change[1]	Net effect on infarct risk[2]
147	1981	20	ad libitum	acute	collagen aggregation	=	0
					ADP aggregation	=	
					bleeding time	=	
148	1982	12	50[3]	acute	bleeding time	=	0
149	1982	12	120	acute	plasma thromboxane	↓	0
					plasma prostacycline	↓	
					ADP-induced thromboxane production	↑	
150	1982	8	120	acute	serum thromboxane	↓	+
151	1983	7	64	acute	adrenaline aggregation	↓	+
					collagen aggregation	=	
					ADP aggregation	=	
					thromboxane production		
					adrenaline-induced	↓	
					collagen-induced	↓	
					ADP-induced	=	

Table 2 (continued)

Ref.	Year of investi-gation	Number of volunteers	Alcohol dose, g	Term	Parameter	Change[1]	Net effect on infarct risk[2]
152	1984	10	51	acute	collagen aggregation	↓	+
					ADP aggregation	↓	
					bleeding time	↑	
153	1984	6	32	acute	plasma prostacycline	↑	+
154	1984	15	100	acute	fasting		+
					collagen aggregation	=	
					ADP aggregation	=	
					after SAFA consumption		
					collagen aggregation	↓	
					ADP aggregation	↓	
					after PUFA consumption		
					collagen aggregation	=	
					ADP aggregation	=	
155	1984	4	32	acute	collagen aggregation	=	0
					ADP aggregation	=	
					thromboxane production	=	
156	1985	8	120	acute	ADP aggregation	↑	–
					thromboxane production	↑	
157	1985	10	120	acute	ADP aggregation	↑	–
					thromboxane production	↑	
158	1987	12	88	acute	ADP aggregation	=	0
					thromboxane production	=	
159	1987	6	20	acute	ADP aggregation	=	0
					thromboxane production	=	
130	1987	12	23 and 46	5 weeks	collagen aggregation	↓	+
					bleeding time	↓	

SAFA = saturated fatty acids; PUFA = polyunsaturated fatty acids.
[1] ↓, decrease; =, no change; ↑, increase.
[2] –, unfavourable effect; 0, no effect; +, favourable effect.
[3] Absolute doses, irrespective of the volunteer's body weight, converted for a hypothetical 80-kg subject for comparison sake.

Stimulation of platelets induces the release of β-thromboglobulin and PF-4. Levels of these proteins in plasma may be indicative of platelet activation in the circulation, provided activation is avoided during blood sampling. To date such analyses have not been taken into consideration in alcohol research.

Only few studies have paid attention to the effects of alcohol on fibrinolytic parameters. Elmér et al. [152] have found effects on bleeding time and platelet aggregation after whisky consumption, but have not found any effects on fibrinolytic parameters. Anderson et al. [162], however, have reported a dose-dependent decrease of fibrinolytic activity after consumption of cider. This finding has been confirmed by Olsen and Østerud [163] for a mixture of pure alcohol and fruit juice. In contrast, in a recent study of Sumi et al. [164] increased fibrinolytic activity was observed 1 h after the consumption of shochu (a spirit), sake and beer. These increases were attributed to a specific urokinase-type plasminogen activator (uk-PA). Pikaar et al. [130] studying the longer-term effects of a dose of 2 and 4 glasses of wine on another activator, tissue-type plasminogen activator (t-PA), have found a dose-dependent decrease. The acute effect of moderate alcohol consumption on t-PA has also been investigated in our study mentioned earlier. One hour after the consumption of 1 glass of port and 2 glasses of wine, in combination with dinner, t-PA was found to have decreased considerably, particularly in middle-aged male subjects [165, 166].

Further research is needed to provide more insight into the net effect of moderate alcohol consumption on fibrinolysis. It is essential that the effects on various fibrinolytic parameters be studied simultaneously.

Summary

The association between alcohol consumption and blood pressure found in epidemiological research has initially been confirmed by experimental studies. However, these studies have not taken the caloric value of alcohol into account. Neither in a study among healthy volunteers nor in a study among CHD patients, in which the acute effects of alcohol intake were measured relative to those of an isocaloric amount of a nonalcoholic beverage, an alcohol-specific increase of blood pressure was found. So far, no well-controlled isocaloric research into the long-term association between alcohol consumption and blood pressure has been carried out.

In many studies an increase of HDL-C level has been found among healthy volunteers after some weeks of alcohol consumption. In some of these studies increases of Apo-A_1 and Apo-A_2 levels have also been observed. There is still some controversy as to the question which HDL-C fraction is increased by alcohol consumption.

Alcoholism has been associated with an increase of HDL-C levels, particularly of the HDL$_2$ fraction. These levels decrease rapidly, within 2 days, upon alcohol abstention. In healthy volunteers a high intake of alcohol (60 g/day) has been found to increase HDL$_2$ levels within 2 days even in the fasting state. The mechanism by which alcohol influences HDL-C levels is still unknown.

Only few studies have paid any attention to the acute effects of a moderate alcohol dose on cholesterol metabolism in the postprandial phase. These effects are still unclear. However, a constant moderate alcohol use might protect against CHD through the reiterative, relatively brief favourable effect on reverse cholesterol transport. This might also explain why the daily intake of a moderate dose of alcohol has a more favourable effect than an irregular drinking pattern.

There is still much uncertainty as to the effects of moderate alcohol use on haemostasis. In some studies a decreased platelet reactivity has been found soon after alcohol ingestion. An increase of the aggregation inhibitor prostacyclin in plasma has also been observed. However, other studies have not confirmed this finding; in contrast, even an increase of aggregation shortly after ingestion of a high alcohol dose (1.5 g/kg body weight) has been reported. Hardly any attention has been paid to the effect of alcohol use over a period of some days or some weeks. In one study aggregation has been found to decrease after consumption of 2 or 4 glasses of red wine a day over a period of 5 weeks, whereas no effect has been found after 4 days.

Fibrinolytic parameters also appear to be affected by alcohol, but the various types of plasminogen activator have been reported to change in the opposite direction.

Final Considerations

Many epidemiological studies have proved that moderate users of alcohol are at lower risk of CHD than teetotallers. In contrast, excessive alcohol use is supposed to increase CHD risk and entails other health risks as well.

Several biological mechanisms could explain the U-shaped relationship between alcohol use and CHD risk. First, there may be a U-shaped or J-shaped connection between alcohol use and blood pressure. Second, alcohol consumption may have a favourable effect on cholesterol metabolism. Third, alcohol has been suggested to affect haemostasis favourably.

Excessive alcohol use, even on an irregular basis, entails increased health risks and is also detrimental in a social context. Measures directed at alcohol moderation, therefore, should aim at driving back alcohol abuse. In contrast, there are, from the viewpoint of health policy, no reasonable arguments for general discouragement or suppression of moderate and sensible alcohol consumption. However, propagation of moderate alcohol use is not free of risk since alcohol consumption even in moderate amounts may be harmful in for example traffic or during pregnancy. Furthermore, it may encourage heavy users to be faithful to their risky habits and moderate users to turn their sensible drinking pattern into a less prudent one. The latter may be especially true for people who are at high risk for alcoholism.

Finally, favourable effects of alcohol use have primarily been observed on a population level and are not necessarily applicable to individuals.

References

1 Brummer, P.: Coronary mortality and living standard. II. Coffea, tea, cacao, alcohol and tobacco. Acta Med. Scand. *186:* 61–63 (1969).

2 St. Leger, A.S.; Cochrane, A.L.; Moore, F.: Factors associated with cardiac mortality in developed countries with particular reference to the consumption of wine. Lancet *i:* 1017–1020 (1979).

3 LaPorte, R.E.; Cresanta, J.L.; Kuller, L.H.: The relationship of alcohol consumption to atherosclerotic heart disease. Prev. Med. *9:* 22–40 (1980).

4 Hegsted, D.M.; Ausman, L.M.: Diet, alcohol and coronary heart disease in men. J. Nutr. *118:* 1184–1189 (1988).

5 Schmidt, W.; Popham, R.E.: Alcohol consumption and ischemic heart disease: Some evidence from population studies. Br. J. Addict. *76:* 407–417 (1981).

6 Stason, W.B.; Neff, R.K.; Miettinen, O.S.; Jick, H.: Alcohol consumption and non-fatal myocardial infarction. Am. J. Epidemiol. *104:* 603–608 (1976).

7 Hennekens, C.H.; Rosner, B.; Cole, D.S.: Daily alcohol consumption and fatal coronary heart disease. Am. J. Epidemiol. *107:* 196–200 (1978).

8 Klatsky, A.L.; Friedman, G.D.; Siegelaub, A.B.: Alcohol consumption before myocardial infarction. Results from the Kaiser-Permanente epidemiologic study of myocardial infarction. Ann. Intern. Med. *81:* 294–301 (1974).

9 Petitti, D.B.; Wingerd, J.; Pellegrin, F.; Ramcharan, S.: Risk of vascular disease in woman. Smoking, oral contraceptives, noncontraceptive estrogens, and other factors. JAMA *242:* 1150–1154 (1979).

10 Ramsay, L.E.: Alcohol and myocardial infarction in hypertensive men. Am. Heart J. *98:* 402–403 (1979).

11 Rosenberg, L.; Slone, D.; Shapiro, S.; Kaufman, D.W.; Miettinen, O.S.; Stolley, P.D.: Alcoholic beverages and myocardial infarction in young women. Am. J. Public. Health *71:* 82–85 (1981).

12 Ross, R.K.; Mack, T.M.; Paganini-Hill, A.; Arthur, M.; Henderson, B.E.: Menopausal oestrogen therapy and protection from death from ischaemic heart disease. Lancet *i:* 858–860 (1981).

13 Kaufman, D.W.; Rosenberg, L.; Hemrich, S.P.; Shapiro, S.: Alcoholic beverages and myocardial infarction in young men. Am. J. Epidemiol. *121:* 548–554 (1985).

14 Barboriak, J.J.; Anderson, A.J.; Hoffmann, R.G.: Smoking, alcohol and coronary artery occlusion. Atherosclerosis *43:* 277–282 (1982).

15 Barboriak, J.J.; Anderson, A.J.; Rimm, A.A.; Tristani, F.E.: Alcohol and coronary arteries. Alcohol Clin. Exp. Res. *3:* 29–32 (1979).
16 Gruchow, H.W.; Hoffmann, R.G.; Anderson, A.J.; Barboriak, J.J.: Effects of drinking patterns on the relationship between alcohol and coronary occlusion. Atherosclerosis *43:* 393–404 (1982).
17 Pearson, TA.; Bulkley, B.H.; Achuff, S.C.; Kwiterovich, P.O.; Gordis, L.: The association of low levels of HDL-cholesterol and arteriographically defined coronary artery disease. Am. J. Epidemiol. *109:* 285–295 (1979).
18 Fried, L.P.; Moore, R.D.; Pearson, T.A.: Long-term effects of cigarette smoking and moderate alcohol consumption on coronary artery diameter. Am. J. Med. *80:* 27–44 (1986).
19 Gordon, T.; Kannel, W.B.: Drinking habits and cardiovascular disease: The Framingham Study. Am. Heart J. *105:* 667–673 (1983).
20 Kannel, W.B.; Castelli, W.P.; McNamara, P.M.: The coronary profile: 12-year follow-up in the Framingham Study. J. Occup. Med. *12:* 611–619 (1967).
21 Colditz, G.A.; Branch, L.G.; Lipnick, R.J.; Willett, W.C.; Rosner, B.; Posner, B.; Hennekens, C.H.: Moderate alcohol and decreased cardiovascular mortality in an elderly cohort. Am. Heart J. *109:* 886–889 (1985).
22 Yano, K.; Reed, D.M.; McGee, D.L.: Ten-year incidence of coronary heart disease in the Honolulu Heart Program. Am. J. Epidemiol. *119:* 653–666 (1984).
23 Yano, K.; Rhodas, G.G.; Kagan, A.: Coffee, alcohol and risk of coronary heart disease among Japanese men living in Hawaii. N. Engl. J. Med. *297:* 405–409 (1977).
24 Blackwelder, W.C.; Yano, K.; Rhoads, G.G.; Kagan, A.; Gordon, T.; Palesch, Y.: Alcohol and mortality: The Honolulu Heart Study. Am. J. Med. *68:* 164–168 (1980).
25 Dyer, A.R.; Stamler, J.; Paul, O.; Lepper, M.H.; Shekelle, R.B.; McKean, H.; Garside, D.: Alcohol consumption and 17-year mortality in the Chicago Western Electric Company Study. Prev. Med. *9:* 78–90 (1980).
26 Klatsky, A.L.; Friedman, G.D.; Siegelaub, A.B.: Alcohol and mortality. A ten-year Kaiser-Permanente Experience. Ann. Intern. Med. *95:* 139–145 (1981).
27 Klatsky, L.; Armstrong, M.A.; Friedman, G.D.: Relations of alcoholic beverage use to subsequent coronary artery disease hospitalization. Am. J. Cardiol. *58:* 710–714 (1986).
28 Cullen, K.; Stenhouse, N.S.; Wearne, K.L.: Alcohol and mortality in the Busselton Study. Int. J. Epidemiol. *11:* 67–70 (1982).
29 Kozararevic, D.; Vojvodic, N.; Dawber, T.; McGee, D.; Racic, Z.; Gordon, T.: Frequency of alcohol consumption and morbidity and mortality: The Yugoslavia cardiovascular disease study. Lancet *i:* 613–616 (1980).
30 Salonen, J.T.; Puska, P.; Nissinen, A.: Intake of spirits and beer and risk of myocardial infarction and death. A longitudinal study in eastern Finland. J. Chronic Dis. *36:* 533–543 (1983).
31 Kittner, S.J.; Garcia-Palmleri, M.R.; Costas, R.; Cruz-Vidal, M.; Abbott, R.D.; Havlik, R.J.: Alcohol and coronary heart disease in Puerto Rico. Am. J. Epidemiol. *117:* 538–550 (1983).
32 Gordon, T.; Doyle, J.T.: Drinking and coronary heart disease: The Albany Study. Am. Heart J. *110:* 331–334 (1985).

33 Marmot, M.G.; Shipley, M.J.; Rose, G.; Thomas, B.J.: Alcohol and mortality: A U-shaped curve. Lancet *i:* 580–583 (1981).

34 Kono, S.; Ikeda, M.; Ogata, M.; Tokudome, S.; Nishizumi, M.; Kuratsune, M.: The relationship between alcohol and mortality among Japanese physicians. Int. J. Epidemiol. *12:* 437–441 (1983).

35 Kono, S.; Ikeda, M.; Tokudome, S.; Nishizumi, M.; Kuratsune, M.: Alcohol and mortality: A cohort of male Japanese physicians. Int. J. Epidemiol. *15:* 527–532 (1986).

36 Greig, M.; Pemberton, J.; Hay, I.; MacKenzie, G.: A prospective study of the development of coronary heart disease in a group of 1,202 middle-aged men. J. Epidemiol. Community Health *34:* 23–30 (1980).

37 Camacho, T.C.; Kaplan, G.A.; Richard, D.: Alcohol consumption and mortality in Almeda County. J. Chronic Dis. *40:* 229–236 (1987).

38 Suhonen, O.; Aromaa, A.; Reunanen, A.; Knekt, P.: Alcohol consumption and sudden coronary death in middle-aged Finnish men. Acta Med. Scand. *221:* 335–341 (1987).

39 Friedman, L.A.; Kimball, A.W.: Coronary heart disease mortality and alcohol consumption in Framingham. Am. J. Epidemiol. *124:* 481–489 (1986).

40 Wolf, P.A.; Kannel, W.B.; Verter, J.: Current status of stroke risk factors. Neurol. Clin. *1:* 317–343 (1983).

41 Shaper, A.G.; Wannamethee, G.; Walker, M.: Alcohol and mortality in British men: explaining the U-shaped curve. Lancet *ii:* 1267–1273 (1988).

42 Alcohol and the U-shaped curve. Lancet *i:* 105 (1989).

43 Alcohol and the U-shaped curve. Lancet *i:* 224–225 (1989).

44 Alcohol and the U-shaped curve. Lancet *i:* 336 (1989).

45 Stampfer, M.J.; Colditz, G.A.; Willett, W.C.; Speizer, F.E.; Hennekens, C.H.: A prospective study of moderate alcohol consumption and the risk of coronary disease and stroke in women. N. Engl. J. Med. *319:* 267–273 (1988).

46 Lian, C.: L'alcoholisme, cause d'hypertension artérielle. Bull. acad. Natl Med. (Paris) *74:* 525–528 (1915).

47 Arkwright, P.D.; Beilin, L.J.; Rouse, I.; Armstrong, B.K.; Vandongen, R.: Alcohol: effect on blood pressure and predisposition to hypertension. Clin. Sci. *61:* 373S–375S (1981).

48 Cooke, K.M.; Frost, G.W.; Stokes, G.S.: Blood pressure and its relationship to low levels of alcohol consumption. Clin. Exp. Pharmacol. Physiol. *10:* 229–233 (1983).

49 Dyer, A.R.; Stamler, E.; Oglesby,P.: Alcohol consumption, cardiovascular risk factors, and mortality in two Chicago epidemiologic studies. Circulation *56:* 1067–1074 (1977).

50 Gordon, T.; Kannel, W.B.: Drinking and its relation to smoking, blood pressure, blood lipids, and uric acid. Arch. Intern. Med. *143:* 1366–1374 (1983).

51 Gyntelberg, F.; Meyer, J.: Relationship between blood pressure and physical fitness and alcohol consumption in Copenhagen males aged 40–59. Acta Med. Scand. *195:* 375–380 (1974).

52 Harburg, E.; Ozgoren, F.; Hawthorne, V.M.; Schork, M.A.: Community norms of alcohol usage and blood pressure: Tecumseh, Michigan. Am. J. Public Health *70:* 813–820 (1980).

53 Klatsky, A.L.; Friedman, G.D.; Siegelaub, A.B.; Gerard, M.J.: Alcohol consumption and blood pressure. N. Engl. J. Med. *296:* 1194–1200 (1977).

54 Myrhed, M.: Alcohol consumption in relation to factors associated with ischemic heart disease. Acta Med. Scand. *195:* suppl., p. 567 (1974).

55 Pincherle, G.; Robinson, D.: Mean blood pressure and its relation to other factors determined at a routine executive health examination. J. Chronic Dis. *27:* 245–260 (1974).

56 Mitchell, P.I.; Morgan, M.J.; Boadle, D.J.: Role of alcohol in the aetiology of hypertension. Med. J. Aust. *23:* 198–200 (1980).

57 Grobbee, D.E.; Hofman, A.: Alcohol en bloeddruk. Ned. Tijdschr. Geneeskd. *129:* 634–638 (1985).

58 Cairns, V.; Keil, U.; Kleinbaum, D.; Doering, A.; Stieber, J.: Alcohol consumption as a risk factor for high blood pressure. Hypertension *6:* 124–131 (1984).

59 Ueshima, J.H.; Shimamoto, Y.; Lida, M.: Alcohol intake and hypertension among urban and rural Japanese populations. J. Chronic Dis. *37:* 585–592 (1989).

60 Harlan, W.R.; Hull, A.L.; Schmouder, R.L.; Landis, J.R.; Thompson, F.E.; Larkin, F.A.: Blood pressure and nutrition in adults. Am. J. Epidemiol. *120:* 17–28 (1984).

61 Gill, J.S.; Zezulka, A.V.; Shipley, M.J.; Gill, S.K.; Beevers, D.G.: Stroke and alcohol consumption. N. Engl. J. Med. *315:* 1041–1046 (1986).

62 Gorelic, P.B.: Alcohol and stroke. Stroke *19:* 268–271 (1987).

63 Hillbom, M.: What supports the role of alcohol as a risk factor for stroke? Acta Med. Scand. *717:* suppl., pp. 93–106 (1987).

64 Carlson, L.A.; Ericsson, M.: Quantitative and qualitative serum lipoprotein analysis. Part 2. Studies in male survivors of myocardial infarction. Atherosclerosis *21:* 435–450 (1975).

65 Castelli, W.P.; Doyle, J.T.; Gordon, T.; Hames, C.G.; Hjortland, M.C.; Hulley, S.B.; Kagan, A.; Zukel, W.K.: HDL-cholesterol and other lipids in coronary heart disease. Circulation *55:* 767–772 (1977).

66 Goldbourt, U.; Medali, J.H.: High-density lipoprotein cholesterol and incidence of coronary heart disease – The Israeli ischemic heart disease study. Am. J. Epidemiol. *109:* 296–308 (1979).

67 Gordon, T.; Castelli, W.P.; Hjortland, M.C.; Kannel, W.B.; Dawber, T.R.: High-density lipoprotein as a protective factor against coronary heart disease. Am. J. Med. *62:* 707–714 (1977).

68 Jensen, G.; Schnohr, P.; Faergeman, O.; Meinertz, H.; Nyboe, J.; Hansen, A.T.: HDL-cholesterol and ischaemic cardiovascular disease in the Copenhagen City Heart Study. Dan. Med. Bull. *27:* 139–142 (1980).

69 Keys, A.: Alpha-lipoprotein (HDL) cholesterol in the serum and the risk of coronary heart disease and death. Lancet *ii:* 603–606 (1980).

70 Miller, N.E.; Thelle, D.S.; Forde, O.H.; Mjos, O.D.: The Tromsø Heart Study. High-density lipoprotein and coronary heart disease: A prospective case-control study. Lancet *i:* 965–967 (1977).

71 Rhoads, G.G.; Gulbrandsen, C.L.; Kagan, A.: Serum lipoproteins and coronary heart disease in a population study of Hawaii Japanese men. N. Engl. J. Med. *294:* 293–298 (1976).

72   Allen, J.K.; Adena, M.A.: The association between plasma cholesterol, high-density lipoprotein cholesterol, triglycerides and uric acid in ethanol consumers. Ann. Clin. Biochem. *22:* 62–66 (1985).

73   Angelico, F.; Bucci, A.; Capocaccia, R.; Morisi, G.; Terzino, M.; Ricci, G.: Further considerations on alcohol intake and coronary risk factors in a Rome working population group: HDL-cholesterol. Ann. Nutr. Metab. *26:* 73–76 (1982).

74   Barboriak, J.J.; Anderson, A.J.; Hoffmann, R.G.: Interrelationship between coronary artery occlusion, high-density lipoprotein cholesterol, and alcohol intake. J. Lab. Clin. Med. *94:* 348–353 (1979).

75   Barboriak, J.J.; Gruchow, H.W.; Anderson, A.J.: Alcohol consumption in the diet-heart controversy. Alcohol. Clin. Exp. Res. *7:* 31–34 (1983).

76   Barrett-Connor, E.; Suarez, L.: A community study of alcohol and other factors associated with the distribution of high-density lipoprotein cholesterol in older vs. younger men. Am. J. Epidemiol. *115:* 888–893 (1982).

77   Brenn, T.: The Tromsø Heart Study: alcoholic beverages and coronary risk factors. J. Epidemiol. Community Health *40:* 249–256 (1986).

78   Castelli, W.P.; Gordon, T.; Hjortland, M.C.; Kagan, A.; Doyle, J.T.; Hames, C.G.; Hulley, S.B.; Zukel, W.J.: Alcohol and blood lipids. The cooperative lipoprotein phenotyping study. Lancet *ii:* 153–155 (1977).

79   Chen, H.; Zhuang, H.; Han, Q.: Serum high-density lipoprotein cholesterol and factors influencing its levels in healthy Chinese. Atherosclerosis *48:* 71–79 (1983).

80   Croft, J.B.; Freedman, D.S.; Cresanta, J.L.; Srinivasan, S.R.; Burke, G.L.; Hunter, S.M.; Webber, L.S.; Smoak, C.G.; Berenson, G.S.: Adverse influences of alcohol, tobacco, and oral contraceptive use on cardiovascular risk factors during transition to adulthood. Am. J. Epidemiol. 126: 202–213 (1987).

81   Diehl, A.K.; Fuller, J.H.; Mattock, M.B.; Salter, A.M.; Gohari, R.E.; Keen, H.: The relationship of high-density lipoprotein subfractions to alcohol consumption, other lifestyle factors, and coronary heart disease. Atherosclerosis *69:* 145–153 (1988).

82   Donahue, R.P.; Orchard, T.J.; Kuller, L.H.; Drash, A.L.: Lipids and lipoproteins in a young adult population. Am. J. Epidemiol. *122:* 458–467 (1985).

83   Ernst, N.; Fisher, M.; Smith, W.; Gordon, T.; Rifkind, B.M.; Little, J.A.; Mishkel, M.A.; Williams, O.D.: The association of plasma high-density lipoprotein cholesterol with dietary intake and alcohol consumption. The Lipid Research Clinics program prevalence study. Circulation *62:* suppl. IV, pp. 41–52 (1980).

84   Gordon, T.; Doyle, J.T.: Alcohol consumption and its relationship to smoking, weight, blood pressure, and blood lipoids: The Albany study. Arch. Intern. Med. *146:* 262–265 (1986).

85   Gruchow, H.W.; Hoffmann, R.G.; Anderson, A.J.; Barboriak, J.J.: Effects of drinking patterns on the relationship between alcohol and coronary occlusion. Atherosclerosis *43:* 393–404 (1982).

86   Hulley, S.B.; Cohen, R.; Widdowson, G.: Plasma high-density lipoprotein cholesterol level. JAMA *238:* 2269–2271 (1977).

87   Hulley, S.B.; Gordon, S.: Alcohol and high-density lipoprotein cholesterol. Causal inference from diverse study designs. Circulation *64:* supp. III, pp. 57–63 (1981).

88   Jacqueson, A.; Richard, J.L.; Ducimetiere, P.; Claude, J.R.: High-density lipoprotein cholesterol and alcohol consumption in a French male population. Atherosclerosis *48:* 131–138 (1983).

89 Kagan, A.; Yano, K.; Rhoads, G.G.; McGee, D.L.: Alcohol and cardiovascular disease: The Hawaiian experience. Circulation *64:* suppl. III, pp. 27–31 (1981).

90 Kuller, L.H.; Hulley, S.B.; LaPorte, R.; Neston, J.; Dai, W.S.: Environmental determinants, liver function and high-density lipoprotein cholesterol levels. Am. J. Epidemiol. *117:* 406–418 (1983).

91 Stamford, B.A.; Matter, S.; Fell, R.D.; Sady, S.; Cresanta, M.K.; Papanek, P.: Cigarette smoking, physical activity, and alcohol consumption: Relationship to blood lipids and lipoproteins in premenopausal females. Metabolism *33:* 585–590 (1984).

92 Taylor, K.G.; Carter, T.J.; Valente, A.J.; Wright, A.D.; Smith, H.J.; Matthews, K.A.: Sex differences in the relationship between obesity, alcohol consumption and cigarette smoking in serum lipid and apolipoprotein concentrations in a normal population. Atherosclerosis *38:* 11–18 (1981).

93 Willett, W.; Hennekens, C.H.; Siegel, A.J.; Adner, M.M.; Castelli, W.P.: Alcohol consumption and high-density lipoprotein cholesterol in marathon runners. N. Engl. J. Med. *303:* 1159–1161 (1980).

94 Williams, P.; Robinson, D.; Baily, A.: High-density lipoprotein and coronary risk factors in normal men. Lancet *i:* 72–75 (1979).

95 Williams, P.T.; Kraus, R.M.; Wood, P.D.; Albers, J.J.; Dreon, D.; Ellsworth, N.: Associations of diet and alcohol intake with high-density lipoprotein subclasses. Metab. Clin. Exp. *34:* 524–530 (1985).

96 Moore, R.D.; Pearson, T.A.: Moderate alcohol consumption and coronary artery disease. A review. Medicine *65:* 242–267 (1986).

97 Miller, N.E.; Bolton, C.H.; Hayes, T.M.; Bainton, D.; Yarnell, J.W.G.; Baker, I.A.; Sweetnam, P.M.: Associations of alcohol consumption with plasma high-density lipoprotein cholesterol and its major subfractions: The Caerphilly and Speedwell Collaborative Heart Disease Studies. J. Epidemiol. Community Health *42:* 220–225 (1988).

98 Phillips, N.R.; Havel, R.J.; Kane, J.P.: Serum apolipoprotein A-1 levels. Relationship to lipoprotein lipid levels and selected demographic variables. Am. J. Epidemiol. *116:* 302–313 (1982).

99 Haffner, S.M.; Applebaum-Bowden, D.; Wahl, P.W.; Hoover, J.J.; Warnick, G.R.; Albers, J.J.; Hazzard, WR.: Epidemiological correlates of high-density lipoprotein subfractions, apolipoproteins A-I, A-II, and D, and lecithin cholesterol acyltransferase. Effects of smoking, alcohol, and adiposity. Arteriosclerosis *5:* 169–177 (1985).

100 DeWood, M.A.; Spores, J.; Notske, R.: Prevelance of total coronary occlusion during the early hours of transmural myocardial infarction. N. Engl. J. Med. *303:* 897–902 (1980).

101 The Steering Committee of The Physician's Health Study. Preliminary report: Findings from the aspirin component of the ongoing Physicians' Health Study. N. Engl. J. Med. *318:* 262–264 (1988).

102 Chakrabarti, R.; Hocking, E.D.; Fearnley, G.R.: Fibrinolytic activity and coronary artery disease. Lancet *i:* 987–990 (1968).

103 Franzen, J.; Nilsson, B.; Johansson, B.W.; Nilsson, I.M.: Fibrinolytic activity in men with acute myocardial infarction before 60 years of age. Acta Med. Scand. *214:* 339–344 (1983).

104 Hamsten, A.; Wiman, B.; de Faire, U.; Blomback, M.: Increased plasma levels of a rapid inhibitor of tissue plasminogen activator in young survivors of myocardial infarction. N. Engl. J. Med. *313:* 1557–1563 (1985).
105 Hamsten, A.; Blomback, M.; Wiman, B.; Svensson, J.; Szamosi, A.; de Faire, U.; Mettinger, L.: Haemostatic function in myocardial infarction. Br. Heart J. *55:* 58–66 (1986).
106 Nilsson, T.K.; Johnson, O.: The extrinsic fibrinolytic system in survivors of myocardial infarction. Thromb. Res. *48:* 621–630 (1987).
107 Arnold, A.E.R.; Simoons, M.L.; Lubsen, J.: Trombolytische therapie van het acute hartinfarct anno 1988. Ned. Tijdschr. Geneeskd. *133:* 341–349 (1989).
108 Meade, T.W.; Vickers, M.V.; Thompson, S.G.; Stirling, Y.; Haines, A.P.; Miller, G.J.: Epidemiological characteristics of platelet aggregability. Br. Med. J. *290:* 428–432 (1985).
109 Meade, T.W.; Chakrabarti, R.; Haines, A.P.; North, W.R.S.; Stirling, Y.: Characteristics affecting fibrinolytic activity and plasma fibrinogen concentrations. Br. Med. J. *i:* 153–156 (1979).
110 Potter, J.F.; Watson, R.D.S.; Skan, W.; Beevers, D.G.: The pressor and metabolic effects of alcohol in normotensive subjects. Hypertension *8:* 625–631 (1986).
111 Ireland, M.; Vandongen, R.; Davidson, L.; Beilin, L.J.; Rouse, I.L.: Pressor effects of moderate alcohol consumption in man: A proposed mechanism. Clin. Exp. Pharmacol. Physiol. *10:* 375–379 (1983).
112 Ireland, M.; Vandongen, R.; Davidson, L.; Beilin, L.J.; Rouse, I.L.: Acute effects of moderate alcohol consumption on blood pressure and plasma catecholamines. Clin. Sci. *66:* 643–648 (1984).
113 Stott, D.J.; Ball, S.G.; Inglis, G.C.; Davies, D.L.; Fraser, R.; Murray, G.D.; McInnes, G.T.: Effects of a single moderate dose of alcohol on blood pressure, heart rate and associated metabolic and endocrine changes. Clin. Sci. *73:* 411–416 (1987).
114 Potter, J.F.; Macdonald, I.A.; Beevers, D.G.: Alcohol raises blood pressure in hypertensive patients. J. Hypertens. *4:* 435–441 (1986).
115 Howes, L.G.; Reid, J.L.: Changes in plasma-free 3,4-dihydroxyphenylethylene glycol and noradrenaline levels after acute alcohol administration. Clin. Sci. *69:* 423–428 (1985).
116 Puddey, I.B.; Vandongen, R.; Beilin, L.J.; Rouse, I.L.: Alcohol stimulation of renin release in man: it relationship to the haemodynamic, electrolyte, and sympathoadrenal responses to drinking. J. Clin. Endocrinol. Metab. *61:* 37–42 (1985).
117 Young, J.B.; Rowe, J.W.; Pallotta, J.A.; Sparrow, D.; Landsberg, L.: Enhanced plasma norepinephrine response to upright posture and oral glucose administration in elderly human subjects. Metabolism *29:* 532–539 (1980).
118 Grollman, A.: The influence of alcohol on the circulation. Q. J. Stud. Alcohol *3:* 5–14 (1942).
119 Puddey, I.B.; Beilin, L.J.; Vandongen, R.: Regular alcohol use raises blood pressure in treated hypertensive subjects: A randomised controlled trial. Lancet *i:* 647–651 (1987).
120 Potter, J.F.; Beevers, D.G.: Pressor effects of alcohol in hypertension. Lancet *i:* 119–122 (1984).
121 Malhotra, H.; Mehta, S.R.; Mathur, D.; Khandelwal, P.D.: Pressor effects of alcohol in normotensive and hypertensive subjects. Lancet *ii:* 584–586 (1985).

122 Kelbaek, H.; Heslet, L.; Skagen, K.; Munck, O.; Christensen, N.J.; Godtfredsen, J.: Cardiac function after alcohol ingestion in patients with ischemic heart disease and cardiomyopathy: A controled study. Alcohol Alcoholism *23:* 17–21 (1988).

123 Kelbaek, H.; Heslet, L.; Skagen, K.; Christensen, N.J.; Godtfredsen, J.; Munck, O.: Hemodynamic effects of alcohol at rest and during upright exercise in coronary artery disease. Am. J. Cardiol. *61:* 61–64 (1988).

124 Hartung, G.H.; Foreyt, J.P.; Mitchell, R.E.; Mitchell, J.G.; Reeves, R.S.; Gotto, A.M.: Effect of alcohol intake on high-density lipoprotein cholesterol levels in runners and inactive men. J. Am. Med. Assoc. *249:* 747–750 (1983).

125 Thornton, J.; Symes, C.; Heaton, K.: Moderate alcohol intake reduces bile cholesterol saturation and raises HDL-cholesterol. Lancet *ii:* 819–821 (1983).

126 Haskell, W.L.; Camargo, C.; Williams, P.T.; Vranizan, K.M.; Krauss, R.M.; Lindgren, F.T.; Wood P.D.: The effect of cessation and resumption of moderate alcohol intake on serum high-density lipoprotein subfractions. N. Engl. J. Med. *310:* 805–810 (1984).

127 Couzigou, P.; Fleury, B.; Crockett, R.; Rautou, J.J.; Blanchard, P.; Lemoine, F.; Richard-Molard, B.; Amouretti, M.; Béraud, C.: High-density lipoprotein cholesterol and apoprotein A1 in healthy volunteers during long-term moderate alcohol intake. Ann. Nutr. Metab. *28:* 377–384 (1984).

128 Burr, M.L.; Fehily, A.M.; Butland, B.K.: Alcohol and high-density lipoprotein cholesterol: a randomized controlled trial. Br. J. Nutr. *56:* 81–86 (1986).

129 Masarei, J.R.L.; Puddey, I.B.; Rouse, I.L.; Lynch, W.J.; Vandongen, R.; Beilin, L.J.: Effects of alcohol consumption on serum lipoprotein lipid and apolipoprotein concentrations: Results from an intervention study in healthy subjects. Atherosclerosis *60:* 79–87 (1986).

130 Pikaar, N.A.; Wedel, M.; van der Beek, E.; van Dokkum, W.; Kempen, H.J.M.; Kluft, C.; Ockhuizen, T.; Hermus, R.J.J.: Effects of moderate alcohol consumption on platelet aggregation, fibrinolysis, and blood lipids. Metabolism *36:* 538–547 (1987).

131 Belfrage, P.; Berg, B.; Hagerstrand, I.; Nilsson-Ehle, P.; Tornquist, H.; Wiebe, T.: Alterations of lipid metabolism in healthy volunteers during long-term ethanol intake. Eur. J. Clin. Invest. *7:* 127–131 (1977).

132 Contaldo, F.; D'Arrigo, E.; Carandente, V.; Cortese, C.; Coltorti, A.; Mancini, M.; Taskinen, M.R.; Nikkilä, E.A.: Short-term effects of moderate alcohol consumption on lipid metabolism and energy balance in normal men. Metabolism *38:* 166–171 (1989).

133 Crouse, J.R.; Grundy, S.M.: Effects of alcohol on plasma lipoproteins and cholesterol and triglyceride metabolism in man. J. Lipid Res. *25:* 486–496 (1984).

134 Glueck, C.J.; Hogg, E.; Allen, C.; Gartside, P.S.: Effects of alcohol ingestion on lipids and lipoproteins in normal men: Isocaloric metabolic studies. Am. J. Clin. Nutr. *33:* 2287–2293 (1980).

135 Moore, R.D.; Smith, C.R.; Kwiterovich, P.O.; Pearson, T.A.: Effect of low-dose alcohol use versus abstention on apolipoproteins A1 and B. Am. J. Med. *84:* 884–890 (1988).

136 Camargo, C.A.; Williams, P.T.; Vranizan, K.M.; Albers, J.J.; Wood, P.D.: The effect of moderate alcohol intake on serum apolipoproteins A-I and A-II. J. Am. Med. Assoc. *263:* 2854–2857 (1985).

137 Välimäki, M.; Nikkilä, E.A.; Taskinen, M.R.; Ylikahri, R.: Rapid decrease in high-density lipoprotein subfractions and postheparin plasma lipase activities after cessation of chronic alcohol intake. Atherosclerosis 59: 147–153 (1986).

138 Johansson, B.G.; Medhus, A.: Increase in plasma alpha-lipoproteins in chronic alcoholics after acute abuse. Acta Med. Scand. 195: 273–277 (1974).

139 Danielsson, B.; Ekman, R.; Fex, G.; Johansson, B.G.; Kristensson, H.; Nillson-Ehle, P.; Wadstein, J.: Changes in plasma high-density lipoproteins in chronic male alcoholics during and after abuse. Scand. J. Clin. Lab. Invest. 38: 113–119 (1978).

140 Devenyi, P.; Robinson, G.M.; Kapur, B.M.; Roncari, D.A.K.: High-density lipoprotein cholesterol in male alcoholics with and without severe liver disease. Am. J. Med. 71: 589–594 (1981).

141 Bell, H.; Strømme, J.H.; Steensland, H.; Bache-Wiig, J.E.: Plasma HDL-cholesterol and estimated ethanol consumption in 104 patients with alcohol dependence syndrome. Alcohol Alcoholism 20: 35–40 (1985).

142 Cushman, P.; Barboriak, J.; Kalbfleisch, J.: Alcohol: High-density lipoproteins, apolipoproteins. Alcohol. Clin. Exp. Res. 10: 154–157 (1986).

143 Taskinen, M.R.; Välimäki, M.; Nikkilä, E.A.; Kurisi, T.; Ehuholm, C.; Ylikahri, R.: High-density lipoprotein subfractions and postheparin plasma lipases in alcoholic men before and after alcohol withdrawal. Metabolism 31: 1168–1173 (1982).

144 Välimäki, M.; Taskinen, M.R.; Ylikahri, R.; Roine, R.; Kuusi, T.; Nikkilä, E.A.: Comparison of the effects of two different doses of alcohol on serum lipoproteins, HDL-subfractions and apolipoproteins A-I and A-II: a controled study. Eur. J. Clin. Invest. 18: 472–480 (1988).

145 Goldberg, C.S.; Tall, A.R.; Krumholz, S.: Acute inhibition of hepatic lipase and increase in plasma lipoproteins after alcohol intake. J. Lipid Res. 25: 714–720 (1984).

146 Franceschini, G.; Moreno, Y.; Apebe, P.; Calabresi, L.; Gatti, E.; Noe, D .; de Fabiani, E.; Zoppi, F.; Sirtori, C.R.: Alterations in high-density lipoprotein subfractions during postprandial lipidaemia induced by fat with and without ethanol. Clin. Sci. 75: 135–142 (1988).

147 Dunn, E.L.; Cohen, R.G.; Moore, E.E.; Hamstra, R.D.: Acute alcohol ingestion and platelet function. Arch. Surg. 116: 1082–1083 (1981).

148 Deykin, D.; Janson, P.; McMahon, L.: Ethanol potentiation of aspirin-induced prolongation of the bleeding time. N. Engl. J. Med. 306: 852–854 (1982).

149 Kangasaho, M.; Hillbom, M.; Kaste, M.; Vapaatalo, H.: Effects of ethanol intoxication and hangover on plasma levels of thromboxane B_2 and 6-keto-prostaglandin $F_{1\alpha}$ and on thromboxane B_2 formation by platelets in man. Thromb Haemost. 48: 232–234 (1982).

150 Kontula, K.; Viinikka, L.; Ylikorkala, O.; Ylikahri, R.: Effect of acute ethanol intake on thromboxane and prostacyclin in human. Life Sci. 31: 261–264 (1982).

151 Mikhailidis, D.P.; Jeremy, J.Y.; Barradas, M.A.; Green, N.; Dandona, P.: Effect of ethanol on vascular prostacyclin (prostaglandin I_2) synthesis, platelet aggregation, and platelet thromboxane release. Br. Med. J. 287: 1495–1498 (1983).

152 Elmér, O.; Göransson, G.; Zoucas, E.: Impairment of primary hemostasis and platelet function after alcohol ingestion in man. Haemostasis 14: 223–228 (1984).

153 Landolfi, R.; Steiner, M.: Ethanol raises prostacyclin in vivo and in vitro. Blood 64: 679–682 (1984).

154 Fenn, C.G.; Littleton, J.M.: Interactions between ethanol and dietary fat in determining human platelet function. Thromb. Haemost. *51:* 50–53 (1984).
155 Galli, C.; Colli, S.; Gianfranceschi, G.; Maderna, P.; Petroni, A.; Tremoli, E.; Marinovich, M.; Sirtori, C.R.: Acute effects of ethanol, caffeine, or both on platelet aggregation, thromboxane formation, and plasma-free fatty acids in human subjects. Drug Nutr. Interact. *3:* 61–67 (1984).
156 Hillbom, M.; Kangasaho, M.; Löwbeer, C.; Kaste, M.; Muuronen, A.; Numminen, H.: Effects of ethanol on platelet function. Alcohol *2:* 429–432 (1985).
157 Hillbom, M.; Kangasaho, M.; Kaste, M.; Numminen, H.; Vapaatalo, H.: Acute ethanol ingestion increases platelet reactivity: Is there a relationship to stroke? Stroke *16:* 19–23 (1985).
158 Hillbom, M.; Muuronen, A.; Neiman, J.; Björk, G.; Egberg, N.; Kangasaho, M.: Effects of vitamin E therapy on ethanol-induced changes in platelet aggregation, thromboxane formation, factor VIII levels and serum lipids. Eur. J. Clin. Invest. *17:* 68–74 (1987).
159 Neiman, J.; Jones, A.W.; Numminen, H.; Hillbom, M.: Combined effect of a small dose of ethanol and 36 h fasting on blood-glucose response, breath-acetone profiles and platelet function in healthy men. Alcohol Alcoholism *22:* 265–270 (1987).
160 James, M.J.; Walsh, J.A.: Effects of aspirin and alcohol on platelet thromboxane synthesis and vascular prostacyclin synthesis. Thromb. Res. *39:* 587–593 (1985).
161 Mehta, P.; Mehta, J.; Lawson, D.; Patel, S.: Ethanol stimulates prostacyclin biosynthesis by human neutrophils and potentiates anti-platelet aggregatory effects of prostacyclin. Thromb. Res. *48:* 653–661 (1987).
162 Anderson, J.A.; Gow, L.A.; Ogston, D.: Influence of cider on the fibrinolytic enzyme system. Acta Haematol. *69:* 344–348 (1983).
163 Olsen, H.; Østerud, B.: Effects of ethanol on human blood fibrinolysis and coagulation. Alcohol Alcoholism, suppl. 1, pp. 591–594 (1987).
164 Sumi, H.; Hamada, H.; Tsushima, H.; Mihara, H.: Urokinase-like plasminogen activator increased in plasma after alcohol drinking. Alcohol Alcoholism *23:* 33–43 (1988).
165 Veenstra, J.; Kluft, C.; Ockhuizen, Th.; v.d. Pol, H.; Wedel, M.; Schaafsma, G.: Effects of moderate alcohol consumption on platelet function, tissue-type plasminogen activator and plasminogen activator inhibitor. Thromb. Haemostas. *63:* 345–348 (1990).
166 Veenstra, J.; te Wierik, E.; Kluft, C.: Alcohol and fibrinolysis. Fibrinolysis *4* (suppl. 2): 64–68 (1990).

Jan Veenstra, MD, TNO-CIVO Toxicology and Nutrition Institute,
Department of Nutrition, PO Box 360, NL–3700 AJ Zeist (The Netherlands)

Simopoulos AP (ed): Impacts on Nutrition and Health.
World Rev Nutr Diet. Basel, Karger, 1991, vol 65, pp 72–98

Dietary Intake and Metabolic Parameters in Adult Men during Extreme Work Load

J. Pařízková, J. Novák

Research Institute for Physical Education, Charles University, and Laboratory of
Clinical Biochemistry and Physiology, Health Center for Champion Sport,
Prague, Czechoslovakia

Contents

Introduction

Dietary intake studies in many sport disciplines have shown differences in various athletes as regards their nutritional status in terms of e.g. relative body weight and/or body mass index, and body composition (i.e. absolute and relative amounts of the lean body mass and of depot fat) [1–3]. Marked differences were apparent between those adapted to different work loads which was due both to selection of particular physiques, and adaptation to various exercises requiring skill, or endurance and/or strength (e.g. gymnasts, runners, and/or weight lifters). The level of the aerobic power [2] and of other parameters such as blood lipids and lipoproteins varied also considerably [4]. Significant differences were observed also in the spontaneous dietary intakes, which concern both energy and individual foodstuffs such as proteins, fats, carbohydrates and also minerals and vitamins [e.g. 5–7]. Nevertheless, marked interindividual variability in dietary intake was always observed among athletes of the same sport discipline and very similar performance level [8, 9]. It did not seem that both selection of certain physique, functional predisposition and adaptation could abolish the interindividual differences among champion athletes as has been observed in normal untrained subjects.

Achieving the limits of athletic performance has become a relatively new trend in sports activities. Triathlon, running 100 miles, 'super iron men' competitions and similar extreme and long-lasting exercises [10–12] have been recently organized in many countries of the world. Such activities have obviously a profound impact on the human organism from many points of view as can be shown by functional, or metabolic, biochemical tests. Possible deteriorating effects were also considered. Optimal dietary strategies have been examined aiming at the achievement of as high as possible performance along with the avoidance of adverse consequences. For this purpose, studies are undertaken under conditions of such competitions in which mostly amateur athletes take part.

Undergoing an extreme work load during the above mentioned competitions offers moreover a very interesting physiological model, and the possibility to study the actual energy balance under conditions of an extreme energy output, as well as the reaction of the human organism reflected by parameters of various character. Only selected subjects predisposed for such a work load seem to be able to undergo successfully extreme training and competitions. There appeared moreover a question whether such work loads and participation in extreme long-lasting exercise will normalize more the above mentioned characteristics concerning the dietary intake and nutritional status.

Several groups of athletes participating in a 24-hour run, and/or triathlon and other extreme competitions were therefore followed and examined from the point of view of physique, body composition, dietary intake, metabolic parameters followed in blood and/or skeletal muscle. During all competitions there was a free choice of various warm and cold dishes and of beverages of all sorts; the competitors were encouraged to bring along their preferred meals, refreshments and drinks. The choice and selection of the ingested food was not decisively influenced, and the diet depended on the liking and habits of the competitors. Some drinks were offered and recommended such as G30, a solution of maltodextrin, etc., and their ingestion was also included in the dietary evaluation.

Twenty-Four-Hour Run

Six healthy adult males, all amateur athletes, participating in a 24-hour run, were followed. This run took place in a village close to Prague in April in a stadium and partly outside of it. Running started at 10 a.m. and continued without major breaks until 10 a.m. next day. The participants occasionally interrupted their run for refreshment, drink, food, etc. They varied broadly in age (table 1) as well as in their life habits (including heavy smoking).

Basic somatic characteristics were measured and evaluated: body height and weight, and sum of ten skinfolds. Body mass index was calculated, and the absolute and relative amounts of depot fat and lean body mass were evaluated using regression equations and tables derived in our previous studies for the Czechoslovak population [1].

Table 1 shows somatic and body composition characteristics. Body mass index and the percentage of depot fat were lower than in untrained men of the normal population of the same age range (International Biological Programme Study) [10], but the percentage of depot fat was larger than in champion long-distance and marathon runners [1, 8, 9].

Figures 1–3 show the changes of speed, oxygen uptake V_{O_2} and of the percentage of V_{O_2max} during the 24-hour run which were ascertained at particular time intervals. Marked decline of all values mentioned above during the last part of the run are apparent [12].

Table 1. Mean ± SD values of somatic and body composition characteristics in the participants of a 24-hour run (n = 6)

	Mean	SD
Age, years	38.55	13.1
Height, cm	175.7	5.0
Weight, kg	67.10	4.57
BMI	21.15	1.51
Fat, %	11.7	1.2
LBM, kg	59.0	4.4

BMI = body mass index: weight (kg)/height (m^2); LBM = lean body mass.

Fig. 1. Running velocity during a 24-hour run (mean ± SD).
Fig. 2. Oxygen consumption (V_{O_2}) during a 24-hour run (mean ± SD).
Fig. 3. The percentage of V_{O_2} max during a 24-hour run (mean ± SD).

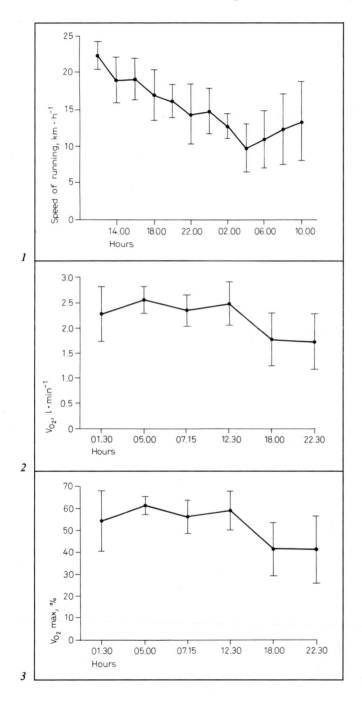

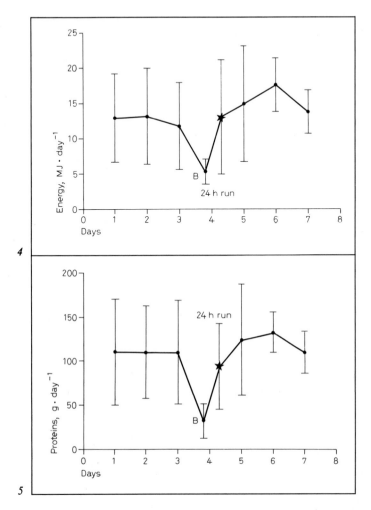

Fig. 4. Energy intake by the participants of a 24-hour run. Mean values (mean ± SD) during the initial, preceding period (days 1–3), at breakfast (B), during a 24-hour run (*) and during the following days (5–7) of recovery are given.

Fig. 5. The intake of proteins before, during and after a 24-hour run (see legend 4).

Dietary intake using an inventory method was followed during 3 days preceding the run; the breakfast just before the 24-hour run was evaluated separately. During the 24-hour run, the athletes recorded their food and beverage consumption, which was on this occasion also checked by an assistant (fig. 4–14). Finally the intake during the 3 following days was also

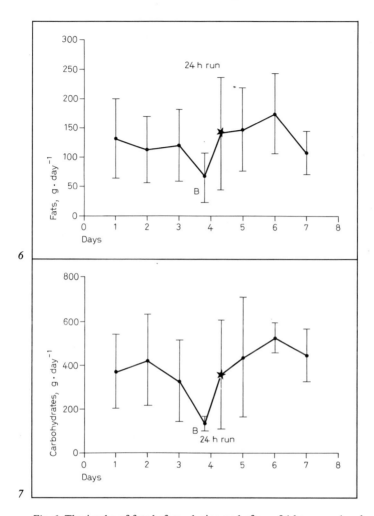

Fig. 6. The intake of fats before, during and after a 24-hour run (see legend 4).

Fig. 7. The intake of carbohydrates before, during and after a 24-hour run (see legend 4).

ascertained. As shown, the individual intakes of energy and of all other items varied markedly.

Spontaneous selection of individual foodstuffs also varied. The intake of proteins before the 24-hour run was 1.5 g/kg body weight, during the run 1.4 g/kg, and during the following 3 days 1.8 g/kg body weight; for fats the

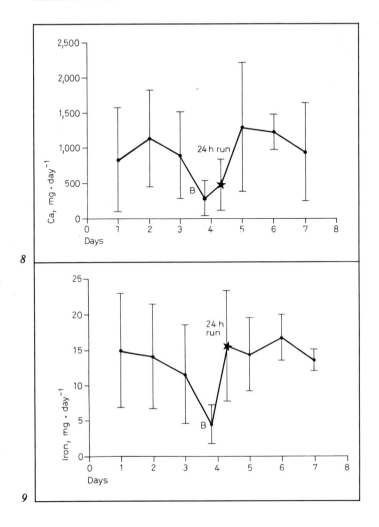

Fig. 8. The intake of calcium before, during and after a 24-hour run (see legend 4).
Fig. 9. The intake of iron before, during and after a 24-hour run (see legend 4).
Fig. 10. The intake of vitamin A before, during and after a 24-hour run (see legend 4).
Fig. 11. The intake of vitamin B₁ before, during and after a 24-hour run (see legend 4).
Fig. 12. The intake of vitamin B₂ before, during and after a 24-hour run (see legend 4).

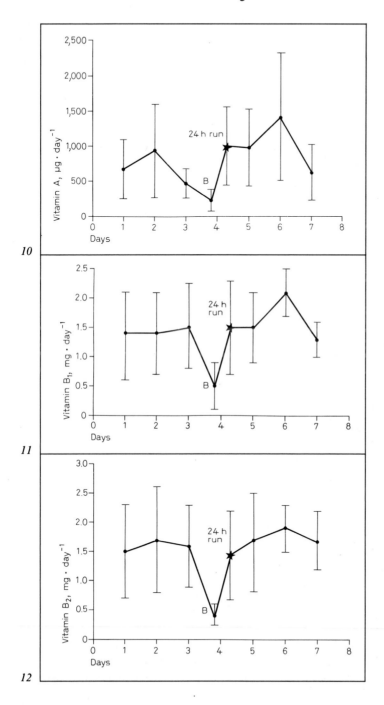

10

11

12

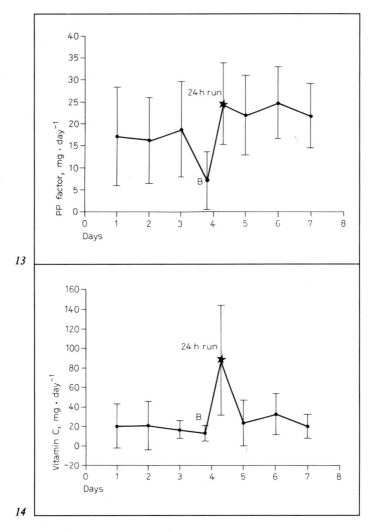

Fig. 13. The intake of PP factor before, during and after a 24-hour run (see legend 4).
Fig. 14. The intake of vitamin C before, during and after a 24-hour run (see legend 4).

mean values were 1.7, 2.1 and 2.1 g/kg body weight; for carbohydrates 5.8, 5.3 and 6.8 g/kg body weight, i.e., the highest values were found during the recovery period. The percentage of energy covered by proteins varied from 12 to 14%, that covered by fats from 35 to 41%, and carbohydrates from 41 to 51%. The percentage of energy covered spontaneously by proteins and carbohydrates was lowest during the day of the run, and that of fats was highest.

The mean value of the distance covered during the 24-hour run was 176 ± 41.5 km. The energy output during the competition was assessed individually from the values of basal metabolic rate (BMR, calculated from body weight by regression equations for individual age and sex categories), and their multiples for the particular performance estimating its character, intensity and duration [11]. During the 24-hour run the energy output was also calculated from the measurements of the oxygen uptake during selected periods of the competition (indirect calorimetry, fig. 2) and the measurements of the speed during the 24-hour run. The mean value of energy expenditure during the 24-hour run calculated with the help of formulas was 52,472 ± 9,137 kJ, but when estimated by indirect calorimetry it was 59,791 ± 11,722 kJ [12].

As can be seen from the values of energy intake and output, there was a marked deficit which was not compensated for even during the 3 days after the competition. The mean values of energy intake during the 24-hour run were practically the same as the recommended dietary allowances for sedentary males of the same age range. The mean energy intake during 4 days after the competition was only slightly increased. Individual values of energy intake and output and/or of the distance covered, did not correlate with energy intake in the diet ingested during and after the 24-hour run [13, 17].

The mean values of RQ ascertained at the same intervals as V_{O_2} varied between 0.79 and 0.87, indicating the utilization of fat. There was a decrease in total body weight after the 24-hour run, but as it was not possible to check exactly the changes of body composition, i.e., especially the decrease of depot fat and/or the changes of hydration of the organism, we may only speculate about the degree of the obvious mobilization and utilization of fat metabolites during the run. The mean values of depot fat in the organism of the runners was, as calculated from the initial values of skinfold measurement, 7.8 kg of fat; this could serve as a source of energy. The level of glycemia remained in the range of normal, or slightly increased values (by ca. 9.5%) during the whole period of the 24-hour run (table 2) [1, 14, 15].

The level of blood lipids, total, HDL- and LDL-cholesterol, Apo-B lipoproteins and of triglycerides decreased during the 24-hour run (table 3). The values of total cholesterol decreased to 89%, that of triglycerides to 24%. the fraction of HDL-cholesterol increased to 121% of the

Table 2. Mean ± SD values of glycemia and blood lactate level at rest, during and after a 24-hour run

		Value[1]					
		1	2	3	4	5	6
Glycemia mmol/l	mean	5.71	5.21	5.70	6.25	6.07	5.69
	SD	1.09	0.64	0.94	0.29	1.18	0.71
Lactate, mmol/l	mean	2.44	1.88	2.16	2.31	2.22	2.17
	SD	0.78	0.55	0.63	0.70	1.31	0.92

[1] Values: 1 = at rest, before the start; 2 = after 3 h run; 3 = after 8 h run; 4 = after 13 h run; 5 = after 17 h run; 6 = after 24 h run; 7 = after 4 days of recovery (in 4 subjects) and after 6 days of recovery in 2 subjects.

initial value, which may be also considered as a positive result of this work load [12–16].

The level of urea increased during the 24-hour run more than twice (by 103%), and that of uric acid by 26.3% of the initial value; this indicates an increased breakdown of proteins and their eventual utilization during this extreme work load. However, 2 days later, levelled to 123% of the initial value and uric acid decreased to 89% of the initial value (table 4) [15–17].

In a parallel study by Macková et al. [18, 19] on the same group of athletes, biopsies from musculus vastus lateralis enabled the evaluation of the distribution of muscle fibers which was similar to typical endurance runners: 59% were slow-oxidative fibers. This corresponded to the values of enzyme activities of energy metabolism at resting condition, e.g. the values for citrate synthetase (CS) and hydroxyacetyl-CoA-dehydrogenase (HAD) activity values were in the range of 0.217–0.267 and 0.140–0.262 $\mu kat/g-1$ w.w. respectively. After the 24-hour run, the activities of enzymes were lowered by 10–87% as compared with initial resting values [18, 19]. The decrease of the activities of hexokinase, lactate dehydrogenase and malate dehydrogenase were statistically significant; on the other hand, as assumed by Macková et al. [18, 19], the smallest changes were found in the activities of enzymes CS and HAD that are usually increased in endurance runners. It is possible to assume that the adaptation to endurance training in these athletes resulted not only in

Table 3. Mean ± values of serum lipids at rest, during and after a 24-hour run

		Value[1]						
		1	2	3	4	5	6	7
Cholesterol	mean	5.13	5.35	5.50	4.87	4.60	4.74	5.16
(total), mmol/l	SD	0.24	0.29	0.50	0.31	0.42	0.39	0.41
HDL-C, mmol/l	mean	1.79	2.23	2.22	2.66	2.61	2.17	1.66
	SD	0.34	0.45	0.57	0.72	0.48	0.42	0.37
LDL, mmol/l	mean	3.01	–	–	–	–	2.46	–
	SD	0.22					0.28	
Index	mean	0.36	0.41	0.41	0.55	0.57	0.46	0.33
	SD	0.03	0.09	0.13	0.17	0.14	0.07	0.09
Triglycerides	mean	1.69	2.11	1.32	1.07	0.65	0.50	1.69
mmol/l	SD	0.49	0.42	0.32	0.32	0.26	0.14	0.64
Apo-B, mmol/l	mean	1.08	1.16	1.18	0.89	0.34	0.74	–
	SD	0.26	0.25	0.20	0.35	0.20	0.27	

[1] Values 1–7 as explained in table 2.

Table 4. Mean ± SD values of urea and uric acid at rest, during and after a 24-hour run

		Value[1]						
		1	2	3	4	5	6	7
Urea, mmol/l	mean	5.82	6.72	8.70	11.40	11.63	11.86	7.18
	SD	1.42	2.43	2.46	2.35	2.75	3.39	1.21
Uric acid, µmol/l	mean	361.3	401.3	461.1	460.5	443.1	456.6	321.0
	SD	72.9	88.9	69.8	69.8	83.0	97.9	54.0

[1] Values 1–7 as explained in table 2.

the increase of the activity of these enzymes (i.e., CS and HAD), but also in the stabilization of their values in spite of an extreme work load [18, 19].

Changes of hematocrit and hemoglobin after the 24-hour run were slight and did not show hemoconcentration, i.e., the drinking regimen during the competition compensated well the losses of fluids from the organism by sweating, etc. [12, 16, 17].

When the mentioned parameters were evaluated after the period of recovery it was shown that most of them returned to the initial values, and the situation of the organism normalized. Therefore, it may be concluded that the adapted organism can tolerate such an extreme work load without any marked consequences. Even when some more marked deviations of normal values occurred, the regulatory mechanisms compensated quite rapidly for such a situation. This was further demonstrated e.g. by only slight changes in the concentration of Na, K, Cl, Mg, and lactate in the blood [12]. In connection with that, it is necessary to stress again that all participants were enthusiastic amateurs and not champion athletes. This study shows furthermore that the dietary and drinking regimens were adequate in spite of large interindividual differences in the dietary intake among runners, differences in the fluctuations of body weight, etc.

No complaints of unpleasant deteriorating feelings were reported by the participants during and after the run. The changes in the lipid metabolism parameters, especially those concerning the decrease of triglycerides and total cholesterol, and the increase in the fraction of HDL cholesterol can be considered beneficial from the health point of view.

Triathlon I

An 'ultraman' triathlon took place in Northern Bohemia during June. It included 10 km of swimming, 100 km of running and 500 km of cycling over a 3-day period (see legend to table 7).

Seven of the participants finished the competition and submitted also in writing down their food intake during the competition and for 3 days under usual life conditions at work, home, etc. Energy, carbohydrate, vitamins etc. content of the beverages consumed during the competition was also evaluated. In this case the age range was smaller (table 5). Somatic characteristics were similar as in the participants of the 24-hour run (table 1).

Actual mean energy intake (fig. 15) was again lower than expected from energy output during the 3-day competition. The intake of proteins, fats and carbohydrates (fig. 16–18) fluctuated slightly during days 1–3. Just at the very end of the period of observation there was some increase of energy intake and of individual food components. It was not possible to

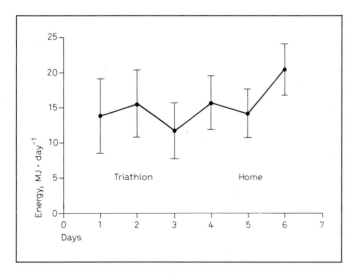

Fig. 15. The intake of energy during 3 days (1–3) of triathlon I and during the days (4–6) following this competition.

Table 5. Mean SD values of somatic and body composition characteristics in the participants of triathlon I (n = 7)

	Mean	SD
Age, years	32.09	7.37
Height, cm	180.0	7.0
Weight, kg	81.4	8.0
BMI	25.1	2.2
Fat, %	10.2	5.6
LBM, kg	73.1	6.8

continue further recording of food intake after the completion of the planned 3-day period. The intake of minerals and vitamins followed the same trend as energy and food intake (table 6) [19, 20].

The values of the intake of proteins as related to body weight varied from 0.8 to 2.2 g/kg body weight, those of fat from 0.91 to 2.18 g/kg, and those of carbohydrates from 5.21 to 6.76 g/kg body weight; lowest relative values (expressed per kilogram body weight) for all these components were found during the last day of the triathlon, and the highest values during the third day after this competition.

The proportion of energy intake covered by proteins varied from 10 to 17%, that by fats from 25 to 35%, and that by carbohydrates from 53 to 61. The lowest values of the percentage of energy covered by proteins and fats were found during the last day of the triathlon, which was accompanied by the highest percentage of energy covered by carbohydrates. The highest value of the percentage of energy covered by proteins was found during the first day after the triathlon, and that for fat during the third day of the period after the triathlon when the percentage of energy covered by carbohydrates was lowest.

Table 6. Mean ± SD values of the intake of mineral and vitamins in the participants of triathlon I (n = 7)

		Day 1	Day 2	Day 3	Day 4	Day 5	Day 6
Minerals							
Ca, mg	mean	952.9	898.8	562.1	1,200.2	1,291.8	1,408.4
	SD	505.9	638.6	251.2	532.0	754.1	1,232.8
Fe, mg	mean	18.3	25.0	10.6	28.7	19.1	23.7
	SD	12.6	17.8	4.2	11.1	6.2	5.2
Vitamins							
A, µg	mean	1,760.1	2,005.7	1,841.5	4,483	1,826.9	1,416.1
	SD	1,059.4	1,561.6	1,798.7	2,373	1,287.4	787.6
B_1, mg	mean	2.4	2.7	1.4	2.6	1.8	2.3
	SD	1.1	0.9	0.6	1.1	0.6	0.3
B_2, mg	mean	3.7	3.4	2.7	3.8	2.1	3.0
	SD	1.3	1.1	1.2	1.3	0.3	0.8
PP, mg	mean	32.7	41.8	29.4	47.1	28.7	47.1
	SD	15.9	11.6	19.2	6.2	8.6	14.8
C, mg	mean	303.1	369.7	209.5	139.2	130.3	139.1
	SD	238.0	229.6	123.4	65.2	60.6	48.7

Fig. 16. The intake of proteins during 3 days (1–3) of triathlon I and during the following days (4–6).

Fig. 17. The intake of fats during 3 days (1–3) of triathlon I and during the following days (4–6).

Fig. 18. The intake of carbohydrates during 3 days (1–3) of triathlon and during the following days (4–6).

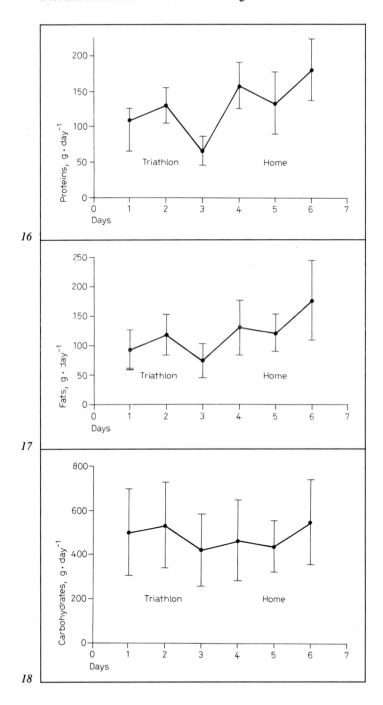

16

17

18

Table 7. Mean ± SD values of serum lipids before and after particular competitions on days 1–3 of triathlon I

		Day 1[1]		Day 2[2]		Day 3[3]	
		b	a	b	a	b	a
Cholesterol	mean	5.11	5.01	4.45	4.72	4.15	4.25
(total), mmol/l	SD	0.70	0.79	0.60	0.86	0.54	0.77
HDL, mmol/l	mean	1.67	1.81	1.96	2.10	1.85	2.05
	SD	0.28	0.19	0.19	0.34	0.28	0.27
Triglycerides	mean	1.57	1.30	0.67	1.08	0.58	0.77
mmol/l	SD	0.68	0.51	0.18	0.13	0.08	0.18
NEMK, µmol/l	mean	0.39	1.14	0.33	1.15	0.29	0.77
	SD	0.31	0.40	0.16	0.24	0.07	0.35

[1] Value before (b) and after (a) 10 km swimming + 200 km cycling.
[2] Values before (b) and after (a) 300 km cycling.
[3] Values before (b) and after (a) 80 km running.

The mean weight decrement after the 3-day competition was 3.6 ± 2.41 kg. The changes in blood glucose levels were within the ranges similar to those during the 24-hour run. The level of total cholesterol in the serum decreased, when comparing the initial and last value by 17%, that of triglycerides by 50% (table 7). On the other hand, the HDL serum level significantly increased by 22% during the same period. Nonesterified fatty acids in the serum (NEMK) always increased after the day's competition; the values on the last day of the triathlon were lower both before and after the days of competition by approximately 33–36% as compared to the values during the first day [22].

Table 8 shows the changes of urea and uric acid. Both of these values always increased after the competition on individual days; when comparing the initial value of urea to the final one the increase was by 43%, and that of uric acid by 30% [22, 23].

These results indicate a similar reaction of the organism to the extreme work load as during and after the 24-hour run. The energy intake was not proportional to the energy output, and even during the 3 days following the triathlon there was no particular increase in food consumption when the competitors pursued their usual professional and leisure

Table 8. Mean ± SD values of urea and uric acid before and after particular competitions on days 1–3 of triathlon I[1]

		Day 1		Day 2		Day 3	
		b	a	b	a	b	a
Urea, mmol/l	mean	7.27	9.14	9.42	12.52	9.35	10.45
	SD	0.91	2.15	1.13	4.56	1.78	2.79
Uric acid	mean	291.86	371.71	320.0	369.67	362.0	381.5
μmol/l	SD	64.86	77.21	68.09	38.93	43.36	47.44

[1] See table 7 for footnotes.

activities. Thus, a marked deficit in the energy balance relative to the actual dietary intake and work output seems to be apparent. There was a marked weight decrement; however, again, it was difficult to evaluate the role played by e.g. depot, endogenous fat in coverage of the energy needs without proper analysis of the composition of the weight decrement. The sum of ten skinfolds did not change after 3 days of competition. Fluid loss could not be entirely evaluated (including sweating, perspiratio insensibilis, etc.).

The changes in serum lipids indicate an increased utilization of lipids as an energy source, especially the increased serum level of nonesterified fatty acids (NEFA) which always increased during the days of the competition; their final value as compared to the initial one increased approximately 97%. The reduction of total cholesterol was similar to that in the 24-hour run. Along with the increased level of HDL (by 22%), a decreased level of triglycerides (by ca. 50%) manifests the positive changes in lipid metabolism during this type of work load.

The changes in urea (an increase by ca. 43%) and uric acid (an increase by ca. 30%) indicate again an increased mobilization of proteins, which might be due to the fact that the actual food intake did not adequately correspond to the actual energy needs. Nevertheless, the daily intake of proteins as mentioned above might be sufficient in the case of an adequately increased energy intake; this was obviously not the case during this triathlon. Protein intake increased during 3 days after the competition to 1.9 g/kg body weight on average as a compensation for the negative nitrogen balance during the competition.

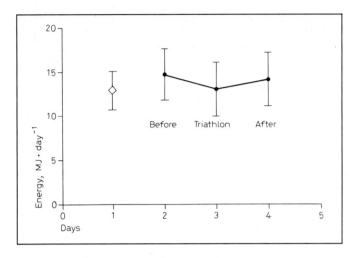

Fig. 19. The intake of energy recorded 3 days before triathlon II (1) and then 1 day before (2), during the day of triathlon (3) and 1 day after it (4).

Table 9. Mean ± SD values of somatic and body composition characteristics in the participants of triathlon II (n = 8)

	Mean	SD
Age, years	26.14	6.66
Height, cm	180.4	3.7
Weight, kg	71.62	5.66
BMI	22.0	1.1
Fat, %	4.9	2.9
LBM, kg	68.1	4.9

Triathlon II

The 'olympic' triathlon (II) was organized in Prague, in which the participants competed in 1.5 km of swimming, 40 km of cycling and 10 km of running over a 2-hour period during one day. Anthropometric and body composition characteristics of the competitors are given in table 9; in this case the competitors were younger and had less depot fat.

Figure 19 shows the energy consumption during 1 day when the competitors were tested in our laboratory; the values show the level of spontaneous energy intake during the day preceding the triathlon II competition, then the consumption during the day of triathlon, and another day following the competition. Figures 20–22 show the intake of proteins, fats and carbohydrates. As can be seen, the intake of energy, proteins and fats was mostly increased during the day of triathlon, which did not apply to carbohydrates. During the day following the competition the intake of energy, proteins and fats, decreased, but the intake of carbohydrates slightly increased.

The intake of proteins related to body weight varied from 1.6 to 1.76 g/kg body weight, that of fats from 1.3 to 1.95 g/kg, and that of carbohydrates from 6.1 to 6.4 g/kg body weight. The proportion of energy intake covered by proteins varied from 14 to 15%, and was highest during the day preceding the competition, and then during the day of triathlon II. The proportion of energy intake covered by fats varied from 27 to 34%, and the highest proportion of energy covered by fats occurred during the last day of the food intake assessment in this group, i.e. 1 day after the triathlon II. Finally, the proportion of energy intake covered by carbohydrates varied from 50 to 58%, and its highest proportion appeared before the competition of triathlon II. As apparent, in the case of triathlon II the variations of the proportion covered by various foodstuffs were smaller as compared to those found during and after large volume triathlon I.

The trend of changes in the spontaneous intake of minerals and vitamins mostly followed the trend of intake of individual foodstuffs with the exception of Fe, and vitamins B_2 and PP factor (table 10).

The evaluation of the energy output based on the WHO [11] again indicated actual energy deficit during the day of triathlon II, which did not seem to be compensated for by the dietary intake during the immediately following day.

'Mount Everest Climbing'

Another extreme work load was undertaken during an imaginary 'Mount Everest climb', i.e., the competition for amateur endurance runners who climbed 80 times up and down during 26.6 h on average a hill in Prague surmounting the altitude of 110 m, with mean resting time 6.9 h. The track distance was 125 km, the slope 8°. Mean speed was 4.7 km/h. The 8 participants (from a total of 14) who sucessfully completed this competition were finally evaluated from the point of view of dietary intake, morphological and biochemical changes during the competition [24].

Anthropometric and body composition characteristics were within the normal range. The initial values of the percentage of depot fat was 10.0% on average, and the aerobic power expressed as the maximal oxygen uptake related to body weight was 53 ml/kg. The values of the weight decrement were 1.5 kg on average. The mean intake of energy during this competition was 21,550 kJ, the mean estimated energy output was 40,450 kJ; the ratio between proteins, fats and carbohydrates was 17:20:63 on average. The deficit between the actual dietary intake and energy output during this work load seemed again marked [2, 24].

The blood level of triglycerides after this competition decreased significantly in the competitors by 60%, that of glucose increased significantly by 17%. The level of urea increased significantly by 48%, that of creatinine

Table 10. Mean ± SD values of the intake of minerals and vitamins in the participants of triathlon II (n = 8)

		Day 1	Day 2	Day 3	Day 4
Minerals					
Ca, mg	mean	1,121.0	1,137.3	758.9	1,294
	SD	816.4	540.6	504.6	577
Fe, mg	mean	16.2	15.7	16.5	16.0
	SD	5.0	4.8	4.6	5.0
Vitamins					
A, μg	mean	1,796	2,350.3	1,191.0	1,738.0
	SD	1,233	1,205.1	692.3	1,012.6
B_1, mg	mean	1.6	1.6	1.6	1.9
	SD	0.5	0.4	0.5	0.8
B_2, mg	mean	2.3	2.5	2.8	2.7
	SD	0.9	0.6	0.8	0.4
PP, mg	mean	25.8	25.8	31.1	27.4
	SD	8.0	7.6	8.4	9.6
C, mg	mean	76.5	138.9	127.1	139.1
	SD	62.3	90.2	104.1	127.3

Fig. 20. The intake of proteins (triathlon II – see legend 19).
Fig. 21. The intake of fats (triathlon II – see legend 19).
Fig. 22. The intake of carbohydrates (triathlon II – see legend 19).

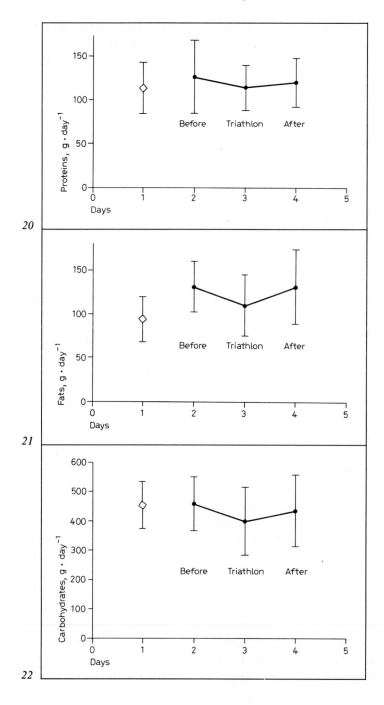

by 32%. Some of these relative changes are similar to those found in previous competitions. The activity of creatine phosphokinase (CPK) increased significantly by 58% [23]. It might be concluded, however, that the amateur competitors were able to undergo without deteriorating consequences such a work load, with an actual energy deficit when comparing the dietary intake and output along with a weight loss, and with positive changes in blood lipids.

The Impact of Very Intensive Training on Cyclists and Marathon Runners

It has been believed that during long-term endurance performance it is necessary to ingest, along with an increased energy intake, also a high amount of proteins. The opinions about the protein intake during endurance loads of an extreme character still vary, starting with normal dietary recommended allowance in the normal range (i.e. 0.8–1.0 g protein/kg body weight) up to highly increased intake (2–3 g/kg body weight); the impact of the high dose was tested in two groups of athletes [25, 26].

Groups of cyclists (n = 26, age 19–21 years, height 176.8 ± 6.6 cm, weight 70.34 ± 8.73 kg, depot fat 5.3 ± 2.31%) and marathon runners (n = 12, age 26.5 ± 3.5 years, height 174.2 ± 3.41, weight 67.87 ± 5.04 kg) were followed longitudinally during training lasting 20 days in cyclists, and 14 days in marathon runners.

Cyclists trained daily during 3 weeks; total distance covered during this period was 2,070 km. Their daily energy intake was 21,788 kJ, with 3 g proteins/kg body weight. The relationship among proteins, fats and carbohydrates was 17:27:56% [25].

After 3 weeks, their body weight and depot fat increased significantly in spite of heavy training (body weight at the end was 70.94 ± 8.49 kg, depot fat was 6.24 ± 2.25%). The serum level of urea (7.69 ± 2.25 µmol/l) and uric acid (267.9 ± 67 µmol/l) increased significantly when comparing the initial and final values (urea 9.85 ± 1.50 µmol/l; uric acid 298.7 ± 65.4 µmol/l). Athletes felt tired, nauseated and their training capacity was limited [24].

Marathon runners were followed during 2 weeks of training when the total distance covered during this period was 333 km. Their daily energy intake was 21,800 kJ. During the initial phase of this study all of them had the same intake of proteins, i.e. 3 g/kg body weight and day. The relationship of proteins, fats and carbohydrates was 17:27:56%. Starting with the ninth day, subgroup L ingested the diet with only 1 g protein/kg body weight; subgroup H continued to ingest the original diet with 3 g protein/kg body weight. The final values of urea, uric acid and ammonia remained the same in subgroup L (urea 6.65 ± 1.46 and 6.53 ± 0.45 mmol/l; uric acid 243.5 ± 110.9 and 249 ± 32.1 μmol/l; ammonia 18.1 ± 5.58 and 19.24 ± 9.58 μmol/l) while in subgroup H they increased significantly (urea 6.48 ± 0.99 and 9.01 ± 0.46 mmol/l; uric acid 325.3 ± 48.6 and 405.7 ± 59.6 μmol/l; ammonia 13.01 ± 3.14 and 26.72 ± 8.27 μmol/l). A decreased intake of proteins during the last 5 days prevented the manifestation of the transient symptoms of pseudouremia. Also the accompanying signs such as increased fatigability, nausea, dizziness and decreased capacity of training were absent in subgroup L of marathon runners [25, 26]. Even when other explanations for the increase of urea, uric acid and ammonia are considered (i.e., an increased breakdown of proteins), it seems to be evident that, in this case, the increased intake of proteins plays an important role in the origin of the pseudouremic syndrome under conditions of satisfactory energy intake (increased body weight and fat). The fad of high protein intake is unjustified and even hazardous. In cyclists moreover, the weight and fat increment shows a uselessly high intake of total energy; the theoretical estimation of energy output and therefore the recommended dietary allowances during the above mentioned cyclist training were overestimated.

Conclusions

When enough energy corresponding to the increase of energy output is available during long-lasting endurance training, increased intake of proteins is not justified, and may be even deleterious. In marathon runners during the above described training, 1 g protein/kg body weight was shown to be fully sufficient. This seemed to apply also to other competitors of extreme work loads; the spontaneous protein intake decreased at the end of the extreme work load, and there appeared increased protein breakdown and actual negative nitrogen balance immediately after the extreme work load. But this seemed to be rapidly recovered during the following period when the spontaneous intake of proteins and of energy increased. The deficit of total energy intake is larger, but may be compensated for over a longer period of time, which was not possible for us to follow.

It would be therefore necessary to study the energy balance over longer periods after competition to evaluate the time necessary to achieve the energy balance. Simultaneously, more exact methods for the evaluation of the immediate changes of total body composition even under field conditions are needed. The composition of the weight decrements from the point of view of the proportion of water, lipids, proteins, etc. after the extreme work loads ought to be evaluated. This would allow us to understand which energy recources – exogenous as well as endogenous – are used, at what proportion and turnover rate, and how all that contributes to the final achievement of the extreme performance.

As is apparent from the present results, selected individuals are able not only to complete the above mentioned extreme work loads successfully, but are also able to recover during a relatively short period without any deleterious effects. In spite of the large actual exogenous energy deficit, the energy needs even during such extreme work loads can be satisfactorily met not only from the relatively limited diet ingested, but also markedly from the endogenous resources, which is indirectly proven by the changes of the lipid or protein metabolic parameters. The ability of sufficient mobilization of necessary fuel for muscle work as well as the aerobic capacity enabling its utilization is one of the most important and essential prerequisites for such a performance.

References

1   Pařízková J: Body fat and physical fitness. The Hague, Nijhoff, 1977, pp 36–47, 197–208.
2   Pařízková J: Age-dependent changes in dietary intake related to work output, physical fitness, and body composition. Am J Clin Nutr 1989;49:962–967.
3   Wilmore JH, Freund BJ: Nutritional enhancement of athletic performance. Nutr Abstr Rev 1984;54:1–16.
4   Tsopanakis A, Tsopanakis C: The lipoprotein ratio in the evaluation of lipid adaptation in elite athletes; in Pařízková J (ed): Nutrition, Metabolism and Physical Exercise. Proc Int Symp in Honour of the 640th Anniversary of Charles University, Prague 1988. Prague, Charles University, 1990, pp 165–178.
5   Åstrand PO, Rodahl K: Textbook of Work Physiology. New York, McGraw-Hill, 1977, pp 449–477.
6   Grandjean A: Macronutrient intake of US athletes compared with general population and recommendations made for athletes. Am J Clin Nutr 1989;54:1070–1076.
7   Van Erp-Baart AMJ, Saris WHM, Binkhorst RA, Vos JA, Elvers JWH: Nationwide survey on nutritional habits in elite athletes. Part I. Energy, carbohydrate, protein,

and fat intake. Part II. Mineral and vitamin intake. Int J Sports Med 1989; 10(suppl 1):S3–S16.

8 Pařízková J: Body composition and nutrition in different types of athlete; in Taylor TG, Jenkins NK (eds): Proc XIIIth Int Congr of Nutrition, Brighton 1985, London, Libbey, 1986, pp 309–311.

9 Pařízková J, Bunc V, Šprynarováš, Macková E, Heller J: Body composition, aerobic capacity, ventilatory threshold, and food intake in different sports. Ann Sports Med 1987;3:171–177.

10 Seliger V, Bartúněk Z: Mean Values of Various Indices of Physical Fitness in the Investigation of Czechoslovak Population Aged 12–55 Years. Prague, Czechoslovak Association of Sports (ČSTV), 1976.

11 Protein and energy requirements. Report of a Joint FAO/WHO/UNU Consultation. Tech Rep Ser 724. Geneva, World Health Organization, 1985.

12 Novák J, Macková E, Bass A, Pařízková J, Heller J, Švarc V, Steinerová A, Macharáček O, Martinča J, Petržílková Z, Stuková YT, Melichna J, Zauner C, Veselková Z, Polívková V: The response to 24 hours running attempt: energetic balance, muscle enzyme activity and biochemical changes in the blood; in Abstr XXIIIrd FIMS World Congress of Sports Medicine, Brisbane 1986, p 200.

13 Novák J, Jeschke J: Extreme endurance performance from the physiological point of vew. I. Functional characteristics of 'super iron men'. Physiol Bohemoslov 1984;33: 549.

14 Steinerová A, Polívková V, Jeschke J, Novák J, Švarc V: Extreme endurance performance from the physiological point of view. II. Changes in lipid and carbohydrate parameters. Physiol Bohemoslov 1984;33:563.

15 Novák J, Švarc V, Steinerová A, Polívková V, Jeschke J, Macharáček O: Extreme endurance performance from the physiological point of view. IV. Changes in blood urea, uric acid, creatinine, creatinine-kinase activity and white blood cell count. Physiol Bohemoslov 1984;33:549–550.

16 Novák J, Macharáček O, Martinča J, Petržílková Z, Macková E, Pařízková J, Heller J, Bass A, Steinerová A, Polívková V, Švarc V, Veselková A, Melichna J, Janák V, Mazurov O: Changes of the selected biochemical parameters in amateur athletes after an extreme work load (in Czech). Lékař a těl vých 1986;14:24–32.

17 Pařízková J: Nutrition, energy expenditure and exercise; in Tsopanakis A, Poortmans J (eds): Physiological Biochemistry of Exercise and Traning, Proc 3rd Int Course, Hellenic Sports Research Institute. Olympic Center of Athens 1987, pp 239–253.

18 Macková E, Melichna J, Novák J, Havlíčková L: A comparison of enzymatic changes and glycogen depletion in skeletal muscle fibres after two different long-lasting work loads. Physiol Bohemoslov 1984;33:544.

19 Macková E, Novák J, Melichna J: Coureurs amateurs de grand fond. Caractéristiques d'un muscle strié (m. vastus lateralis) et réponse du métabolisme énergetique musculaire lors d'une course durant 24 heures. Med Sport 1989;63:3–10.

20 Pařízková J: The evaluation of the dietary intake of various athletes with the help of computers; in Feldkoren BI, Shishina NN (eds); (in Russian). Leningrad, Leningrad Research Institute for Physical Education, 1989, pp 96–104.

21 Pařízková J: Body composition and dietary intake in athletes of different age, sex, performance capacity and specialization; in Bachl N (ed): Advances in Ergometry. Proc 6th Int Semin on Ergometry, Vienna 1989, in press.

22 Novák J, Macharáček O, Racek J, Holeček V: Pathophysiology of large volume triathlon. I. The characteristics of the performance and the utilization of substrates; in Janoušek V, Špála M (eds): Proc Congr on Present Trends in Pathological Physiology (2), Prague, Charles University, 1989, pp 299–300.

23 Macharáček O, Holeček J, Racek J, Novák J: Pathophysiology of large volume triathlon. II. The changes of the activity of kidneys and proteinuria; in Janoušek V, Špála M (eds): Proc Congr on Present Trends in Pathological Physiology (1). Prague, Charles University, 1989, pp 252–254.

24 Bartúňková S, Havlíčková L, Ježek P, Pařízková J: Drinking regime during an extreme endurance load; in Pařízková J (ed): Nutrition, Metabolism and Physical Exercise, Proc Int Symp in Honour of the 640th Anniversary of Charles University, Prague 1988. Prague, Charles University, 1990, pp 239–245.

25 Poslušný Z: The impact of dietary intake on the level of urea, uric acid and ammonia in the serum in cyclists and marathonists (in Czech). Teorie Prax těl Vých, in press.

26 Brodan V, Poslušný Z: The metabolism of proteins and physical work load (in Czech). Teorie Praxe těl Vých Sportu 1981;29:501–504.

J. Pařízková, DrSc, VÚT, Charles University, Újezd 450, CS–11807 Prague 1 (Czechoslovakia)

Simopoulos AP (ed): Impacts on Nutrition and Health.
World Rev Nutr Diet. Basel, Karger, 1991, vol 65, pp 99–123

The Impact of Agricultural Projects on Food, Nutrition and Health

T.A. Brun, C. Geissler, E. Kennedy

Division of Nutritional Sciences, Cornell University, Washington, D.C., USA

Contents

Impact Evaluation: Rationale and Problems

Agricultural development programs have the explicit or implicit aim to improve either the nutritional status of rural families, or farmers' incomes, or the availability of a specific crop. Ultimately agriculture programs that really concern development must have a positive impact on the provision of basic needs for direct recipients and for the region or country. One of the most fundamental of the basic needs is adequate nutrition and this is therefore a closer indicator of real social development as opposed to aggregate indicators of economic development such as growth of agricultural production and GNP. Many programs which are included under the title of agricultural development merely produce greater profits from agriculture for a small minority of national or foreign entrepreneurs and can have a detrimental effect on genuine social development.

There is therefore a need for better evaluations of the impact of agricultural development programs on nutrition and a better formulation of the methodologies required to do so. These methodologies need to be worked out at both the conceptual level and the technical. The conceptual framework needs to include: (1) the impact on the nutritional status of the direct beneficiaries of the programs; (2) the impact on the population not directly benefitting; (3) the mechanisms by which these effects can be explained such as: the food intake of the beneficiaries and on nonbeneficiaries; environmental health; production and income; prices of food, other consumables, land and agricultural inputs; and employment and land tenure.

Secondly within this framework there is a need for the techniques that can be used for evaluation to be refined so as to ideally provide an accurate, rapid, sensitive but, simple diagnostic system that could be widely used.

Thirdly there is a need to understand not only the obvious value of such evaluations for agricultural planning but also the reluctance to carry out, and resistance against, such evaluations that are likely to be encountered, so as to be better prepared to overcome them.

In the late 1940s, the United States, and later several European nations, embarked on a large-scale effort to assist developing countries in increasing their agricultural production and in eliminating hunger and malnutrition. It was assumed that the transfer of western agricultural expertise to the traditional farming systems of developing countries would inevitably result in an improvement in the standard of living of millions of poor farmers. Development agencies had such a deeply rooted faith in the intrinsic value of technology transfer from industrialized to poor nations that little effort was made to monitor the effects of aid programs.

However, after several decades of assistance, many development specialists have become disappointed by the lack of progress in improving living standards in countries and regions where numerous agricultural interventions, such as extension services, subsidies on the import of fertilizers and pesticides, the construction of roads and irrigation canals, and various commercial farming practices have been introduced.

In the absence of formal evaluations using reliable indicators[1], it is exceedingly difficult to distinguish changes attributable to the global economic context from those resulting from development assistance. Therefore, little is known about the effectiveness of individual agricultural projects.

The disillusionment created by the stagnation or even deterioration of the standard of living in a number of heavily assisted areas or countries has promoted interest in the evaluation of the food, nutrition, and health impacts of agricltural projects [28, 31]. Planners now realize that many development projects do not fulfill their publicized aims and that appropriate monitoring of their impacts could lead to an improvement in their structure and implementation. Such work could particularly benefit the most deprived segments of populations.

Aid agencies require assistance in evaluating projects, but there is a dearth of nutrition researchers with adequate field experience and knowledge of appropriate evaluation methodology and the wide array of relevant tools. Some institutions such as the International Food Policy Research Institute (IFPRI) have focused their attention on the design of adequate models to identify the relationship between key determinants of nutrition and health status [19]. A number of researchers have used a variety of techniques of nutritional evaluation, but generally with a very limited number of indicators. The need for rapid appraisal often leads to the sole use of height and weight of children (anthropometric data) to measure nutritional status in relation to socioeconomic factors. While recognizing the usefulness of this type of indicator, it cannot successfully be used to assess a range of beneficial or detrimental effects of rural development projects.

There is a vast array of other available techniques to assess the impact of economic development on nutrition and health, including measurements of growth and body fat; mortality and morbidity statistics; food intake, habits, beliefs and preferences; nutrient content of the customary diet; toxicity and digestibility of food; physical fitness, energy expenditure

---

[1] In this context, an indicator is something which can be measured in order to assess something which cannot be measured. For example, blood pressure or blood hemoglobin are health indicators; income is an indicator of the standard of living.

and physical performance; mental development; birth weights, breast milk output and child development; clinical nutritional deficiency signs and symptoms; blood levels of nutrients and immunological factors; nutrient turnover; hormone levels; and parasite infestation and bacteriological contaminations. Most of these parameters and many others can be accurately measured, but at times their physiological interpretation can be difficult. For example, hemoglobin or seasonal body weight can be precisely quantified and compared to current standards but it is still not clear whether or not a slightly lower hemoglobin or a slight weight loss affects work capacity, resistance to infection, or other physiological functions. Therefore, the selection of appropriate indicators and their interpretation requires a good understanding of their physiological meaning.

Until recently, one factor which has contributed to the inadequacy of evaluation methods is the lack of strong support and encouragement from development agencies. Although these agencies advocated methodology development, they also saw the risks of being criticized for not achieving their stated goals. Researchers designing project evaluations tend to assume naively that evaluation is actually desired by planners, development specialists, politicians, donor agencies, and others involved in third world development. This is not always the case.

It must be kept in mind that evaluation can result in conflicts of interest between those that play various roles in the design and implementation of the project. Results can be used for or against special interest groups such as land owners, local and foreign technicians, administrators, politicians, and aid agencies or to fan rivalries between ministers or ministries. Therefore, although evaluations are generally strongly advocated on paper by development agencies, in practice they have actually often been discouraged or limited to project components that cannot directly affect institutions involved in project management.

The term, 'evaluation of nutritional impact' is not clear to many project leaders because, traditionally, evaluations are not impact-oriented but process-oriented. That is, they examine whether programs and plans have been executed and services delivered within a certain budget and on time. These evaluations are made for the benefit of the funding agency but tell very little if anything about the physical, social and economic effects on the target population. The favoring of process evaluation rather than impact evaluation is due to two factors: the design and data collection is much simpler; the results are much less controversial and less politically charged.

Until recently, scant attention has been paid to the expectations of the potential beneficiaries which should be a key element of the evaluation. Usually only local representatives and higher government officials are consulted, and little is known, in general, about the most deprived segments of the target populations, including small farmers, landless laborers, migrant workers, and ethnic minorities. Only recently have leading development agencies such as the World Bank and the Food and Agricultural Organization (FAO) of the United Nations (UN) recognized the possibility that the nutritional status of some sections of the target population can actually be worsened by development interventions.

It is not always clear whether inappropriate evaluation is due to willful or inadvertent neglect on the part of the development agency. If it is inadvertent, then improved evaluation methods should lead to reorientation of projects to the benefit of the most deprived. However, projects that pay only lip service to alleviating deprivation will resist reorientation even following such an evaluation. For example, in a World Bank project in Puno area in Peru [14], the recommendation of nutritionists from another UN agency that the project be modified to permit 'more equitable participation and distribution of the benefits' among low income farmers was rejected by the agricultural economist. The economist's justification was that the proposed change would push the rate of return below the minimum level needed to justify the project. This example illustrates the observation that evaluation criteria that are acceptable to the funding agencies, depend on the fundamental issue of the view of that agency as to whom the project should benefit first.

Many so-called development projects, if closely analyzed, are not designed for the poor, except possibly through a theoretical trickle down effect. For more than 10 years the Division of Nutrition and Food Policy of FAO has attempted to include nutritional considerations in agricultural development projects. This objective, if successfully implemented, would lead inevitably to new evaluation strategies which would place nutritional status improvement as a major goal of many development projects. In five of the six projects reviewed by Lunven [23], benefits were found to be concentrated in the better-off farms. Lunven, who is the Director of the Nutrition and Food Policy Division at the FAO, expressed his concern that the improvement of the food situation was not given the degree of priority it deserves. In one case in Africa, irrigation development was concentrated, 'in the subregions of the project area that had the best soil, the closest access to water, the most innovative people, and the lower risk of poverty and malnutrition'. In the case of another African project, 'most of the work is concentrated in the central part of the region – the area least affected by severe climatic conditions, poverty, and malnutrition – and [the project is] awaiting yet to be extended to the most seriously affected areas'. Lunven also describes an Asian dairy scheme in which, 'the landless, who make up a large part of the population and suffer most from poverty and malnutrition, cannot benefit from the project', they have no land and therefore have nowhere to graze cattle. Again, if nutritional objectives had been given due consideration, the benefits of the project would have been extended to the more deprived areas.

Because many agricultural development projects do not aid the segments of the population that are most exposed to malnutrition, it is imperative that researchers committed to real development, develop efficient low-cost methods to collect pertinent baseline data on the prevalence of malnutrition in the project area. The availability of this type of information will give strength to the real development lobby to counter the type of projects that have ignored rural poverty, either willfully or by negligence.

In the 1960s and most of the 1970s, development agencies operated in an atmosphere of relative abundance and little scrutiny from donor countries and the public, this situation changed dramatically in the 1980s. Restriction of development loans, the considerable burden of foreign debt in many developing nations, the multiplication of nongovernmental organizations expressing directly the concerns of a larger public for a more rapid elimination of hunger mitigate for more rigorous project design and implementation and the systematic evaluation of the effect of projects on health and nutrition.

Case Studies of Project Evaluations That Assess Impacts on Food Availability, Nutritional Status, and Health

In this section, we summarize nine case studies that have measured or assessed the impact of an agricultural intervention on food availability, nutritional status, or health. These interventions ranged from irrigation projects to the introduction of hand pumps. Our purpose is to illustrate the range of methods, including design and the use of various biological and social indicators, that were measured during project evaluations. This is not an exhaustive review, but rather is meant to illustrate a number of attempts, their strengths and limitations, and to stimulate further analysis of the relevance of these methods in the evaluation of project impacts.

Pilot Rapid Evaluation Study of an Irrigation Scheme in the Lower Plain of Gonaives in Haiti

Our first example is a pilot study to test a method of rapid evaluation of nutrition impact in Haiti. The method was based on an in-depth comparison of a small number of project beneficiaries and nonbeneficiaries selected from the project area and an adjacent control area. The project was a large irrigation scheme, l'Organisme de Développement de la Basse Plaine de Gonaives (ODPG) [8].

This project, initiated in 1972 with FAO assistance, covered 2,750 ha cultivated by families that included about 20,000 people. The information collected by FAO during project preparation indicated that a contiguous control area was similar to the project area prior to initiation of the pumping scheme. Before the implementation of the project, less than one fourth of the land was seasonally irrigated with river water by ODPG. The project installed water-pumping stations and brought a large faction of the area under permanent irrigation. Crops were drastically modified once secure underground water supplies were pumped to farmers' fields with project assistance. Farmers in the project area were, on average, able to irrigate 60% of their land the year round. Cotton, previously a compulsory but low-profit crop, and traditional sorghum areas were decreased, while plantings of corn, beans, eggplant, banana, rice and high-profit vegetables were increased. The new cropping patterns doubled the economic return per hectare. As a result, households in the project area had family incomes 37% higher than in the control area.

Ten households in the ODPG area and ten in a similar ecosystem outside the ODPG area were selected for nutrition and health evaluation. A variety of tools were used, including socioeconomic questionnaires on production and budget, family food consumption, and individual food intake of 1 adult and 1 child per family over 1 week. Anthropometric parameters were measured on an extended sample of adults and children (426 persons), and health and nutrition practices related to disease and weaning were also recorded. Blood hemoglobin level (213 individuals) and parasite infestation (143 individuals) were also measured [8].

Among the changes brought by the project, it was noted that livestock production (mostly cows) had declined because the new cropping patterns reduced forage availability. Animal production in the ODPG area represented only 3.7% of household income compared to 10.5% in the control area. A larger portion of children consumed either fresh milk or powdered milk in the control area, and weaning occurred at a later age than in the project area. Higher fresh milk intake in the control area most likely resulted from the larger number of cows. Absolute wages from agricultural and other employment and their percentage of total income was significantly higher in ODPG households compared to the control households. Land had become so expensive in the project area, that servants and laborers who in the past could plan to buy land, no longer had access to it. The large traditional families (Lakou) tended to split into smaller production units, and polarization developed between commercial producers and landless laborers.

Individual daily energy food intake calculated from food consumption, which was carefully weighed for 1 adult male and 1 child (between the 3 and 6 years of age) for a whole week, was low or very low in both areas, but generally lower in the control area. However, no difference in anthropometric status was found between the two groups of children. Mean hemoglobin levels in both groups of children (0–6 years) were equally low in both areas (8.7 ± 1.45 g/100 ml) compared to the 11 g and more accepted as normal values; mean hematocrit levels were also low and similar in both areas. No positive nutritional effect from the project was apparent.

One third of the children in both areas had eggs of intestinal parasites (*Ascaris lumbricoides*, *Trichuris trichiura* or *Necator americanus* or a combination). By contrast, more than twice as many adults (74%) in the ODPG project area had parasites as in the control zone (28%). The extension of irrigation in the project area was apparently helping to disperse human excreta in the fields, disseminating parasites over vegetables, tools and hands of the laborers; hence leading to a higher prevalence of water-borne parasites.

The general conclusion from this pilot evaluation study was that a very significant increase in household production, income, housing standards and literacy rate occurred as a result of the project. However, despite a significant increase in mean annual family food purchases in the project area (US$ 620) compared to the control area (US$ 440), no beneficial effects on food consumption and nutritional status of adults and children in the project area were demonstrated. This may have been due to the failure of increased food expenditure to provide improved nutritional intake, possibly because of the deleterious environmental effect of the project area counteracting any nutritional improvement. However, the methodology tested may have been inadequate in sample size and the anthropometric and hematologic indicators used insufficiently sensitive.

This example illustrates first the need to study fairly large samples of recipients and nonrecipients in order to be able to identify significant differences of nutritional interest. It also points to the need for a clear understanding of the key factors affecting the nutritional status in conducting the evaluations. Although the project managers were favorable to evaluation of nutritional impact, they had not included any monitoring components in the project design. The evaluation was therefore severely limited by the lack of baseline nutritional information.

Nam Pong Water Resource Development Project in Northeast Thailand

Sornmani et al. [27] compared the socioeconomic and nutritional status of populations living in an irrigated resettlement area, around a man-made lake, and in proximate traditional villages taken as 'control' areas. The basis for comparison included anthropometric measurements, blood biochemical assays to assess vitamin status, and stool examination for parasite infestation.

The irrigation area covers about 13,500 ha, with 3,500 farms in 33 villages. A 400-km^2 lake created by the dam forced the resettlement of villagers whose land was flooded. On the lake side, approximately 60 fishing villages were created and fish consumption increased.

The evaluation showed that few children suffered from obvious signs of malnutrition, but there were no significant differences in these signs between the control and resettlement areas. However, in the irrigated area, children were generally more anemic than in the control area. No differences in the prevalence of thiamine and riboflavin nutritional deficiencies were detected between the two areas.

The authors [27] concluded that the water resource development project markedly improved the socioeconomic status of the people in the project area, especially in the irrigation scheme and in the fishing villages. As in the Haitian case, despite a significant rise in household income, the health and nutritional status of the project and control areas appeared to be virtually the same.

This study demonstrates once more that increased income does not necessarily lead to improved nutrition and therefore development indicators that are limited to only economic measures such as income cannot be used as a proxy for the health impact of a project.

Eradication of Severe Vitamin A Deficiency in Cebu Island in the Philippines

This example describes the impact of a public health and horticultural program designed to increase beta-carotene consumption and eliminate xerophthalmia [26]. This program, launched on Cebu Island in the Philippines, was part of a larger project that compared the relative effectiveness of three separate programs designed to eradicate severe vitamin A deficiency. The three programs included the following:

(1) Public health and horticultural intervention. This program included the provision of medical care, environmental sanitation, deworming, immunization, nutrition and health education, and the establishment of a village cooperative pharmacy. The horticultural aspect of the program consisted of encouraging and assisting villagers in the production in home gardens of vegetables and fruits with a high beta-carotene content.

(2) The universal distribution of vitamin pills. This massive intervention program consisted of distributing vitamin A and E capsules to all children every 6 months.

(3) Vitamin fortification. This program involved the weekly distribution of vitamin A fortified monosodium glutamate (MSG) (used as a flavoring agent) packets. A survey showed that more than 94% of all children consumed MSG more than once a week.

Significant nutritional changes were observed, but not the expected increase in vitamin A status. The mean serum vitamin A level, a good indicator of the risk of vitamin A deficiency disease, was not significantly altered following the public health and horticultural intervention or vitamin A capsule distribution. However, it rose significantly with the distribution of vitamin A fortified MSG. The public health and horticultural program was the most expensive and the least effective in reducing the incidence of avitaminosis A [25]. It is, however, unfair to directly compare the three programs on their vitamin A impact alone. The public health and horticultural program would be likely to produce a variety of benefits (education, nutritional awareness) over a much longer period than fortification or capsule distrubution. In actuality, significant improvements in growth and a reduction in third-degree malnutrition were observed in the public health and horticultural program areas. In addition, hemoglobin levels increased while they decreased in participants in the other two programs. This example shows that projects which had been expected to improve one nutritional issue might have a more significant impact on another nutritional or health-related problem. Therefore, too narrow an evaluation of only the indicators of the nutritional problem directly targeted could miss other aspects of nutritional impact.

This example also illustrates the feasibility and effectiveness of the elimination of vitamin A deficiency by simple interventions. As the authors themselves point out, the health and horticultural program had a broader and longer lasting effect on the subject population than did the other programs. Therefore, evaluations should be implemented in such a way as to identify both short-term and longer-term effects. This is not often feasible due to limitations of funding, but should be encouraged whenever the projects permit.

Plan Chontalpa for Export Crop Production in Tabasco, Mexico

The long-term effects of projects have sometimes been assessed: a classical case study of the impact of agricultural development on child malnutrition is described by Hernandez and Hidalgo [17], which was one of the earliest studies on the effects of export crop production on nutrition. A community in Mexico was studied in 1958 prior to the introduction of Plan Chontalpa (a new agricultural scheme involving cash crops). In 1971, 13 years after project implementation, the authors reported that there was no significant decrease in second- and third-degree preschooler malnutrition as measured by changes in weight for age ratios between 1958 and 1971. Therefore, they concluded that economic gains in the area did not translate into nutritional benefits. However, the findings are somewhat inconsistent. For example, while second- and third-degree malnutrition did not decline, infant and child mortality rates did significantly drop between the two time periods. It is plausible that malnourished children who would have died in 1958 were kept alive in 1971, contributing to the unchanged rates of second- and third-degree malnutrition.

In addition, in comparing the effects before and after Plan Chontalpa, the authors assumed that no other changes besides the project took place in the community over the 13-year period. Clearly, the health and nutritional status of the community could have been affected by a variety of other nonagricultural factors. Without accounting for other potential exogenous factors, it is difficult to interpret the dietary and anthropometric data as presented by Hernandez and Hidalgo [17].

Dewey [12, 13] conducted a different study of Plan Chontalpa to assess its effect on the diet and nutritional status of 149 preschoolers. Families with at least one child 2–4 years old were randomly selected from three groups: (1) households participating in Plan Chontalpa; (2) nonparticipating households in the Plan area; (3) nonparticipating households outside the Plan area. Anthropometric and dietary data were collected for each child. Results indicate that there were no significant differences for any of the nutritional status measures between plan members and non-members in the same area. Dewey concluded that the agricultural plan did not succeed in improving the nutritional status of the region's children.

Dewey used multivariate analysis, a mathematical tool relating plausible causes (such as income) to their effects, to try to explain factors influencing nutritional status. For the children of families participating in the Plan there was no significant correlation between income and any of the measures of nutritional status. Clearly a factor other than income was accounting for the growth of children in the Plan. However, for nonparticipating preschoolers from the Plan area, there was a significant and positive correlation between nutritional status and per capita income; as income increased, nutritional status improved. In contrast, in the non-Plan area (Teco), income was negatively correlated with nutritional status as indicated by weight, weight for height, and head circumference. Dewey interpreted this finding to mean that the rise in income in Teco was offset by higher food prices, and thus preschool nutritional status actually deteriorated. The disparity of findings on the relationship between income and nutritional status raises the possibility that the processes influencing the preschooler's growth may have varied across the three groups. The data do not clearly elucidate this process. It also illustrates the great difficulty of identifying the causes of observed changes or differences between groups. Such multivariate analysis can offer only suggestions of causes rather than firm conclusions, but the use of a wide range of socioeconomic and biological variables specifically chosen for the local conditions is likely to provide stronger explanations of an impact or lack of impact.

Cash Cropping in Kenya

This example shows the weakness of comparisons between areas made at a specific point in time without adequate baseline data to demonstrate that the areas are comparable. A study [18] in Kenya assessed the impact of cash cropping on the nutritional status of preschoolers. Data from the second Integrated Rural Survey were available for approximately 1,400 preschoolers under the age of 5. Initial analyses showed that children from farm holdings that produced commodities mainly for sale were less severely malnourished (defined as either weight for height less than 80% of standard or height for age less than 90% of standard) than were children from subsistence and semisubsistence farms. However, this analysis did not differentiate between food and nonfood cash crops. Additional analyses were performed to distinguish between five cash crops: coffee, tea, pyrethrum, sugar, and cotton. Anthropometric data for children from cash-cropping households were compared with data from children living in the same ecological zone but whose parents did not cash crop. Results indicated that, contrary to the author's expectations, cotton and pyrethrum cultivation were not associated with higher preschooler malnutrition. Sugar production, on the contrary, was significantly associated with increased rates of stunting (low height for age) in one of the two areas studied. Coffee and tea production were not associated with a consistent pattern of preschooler malnutrition. Of the three tea areas surveyed, there was a significantly lower rate of stunting in one, the second was neutral, and the third had a significantly higher prevalence of low height for age.

There are, however, major problems with this type of analytical approach. First, as with most 'cross-sectional studies', that is, studies comparing groups at the same point in time, there is no clear indication that the baseline nutritional status of participating and non-participating households was similar prior to participation in the cash-cropping scheme. As a result, many alternative explanations besides cash cropping could account for observed differences in nutritional status. In addition, samples sizes were small in many of the groups.

What is interesting about the Kenya study is that there is no consistent relationship between individual cash crops and preschool nutritional status. This indicates that the mechanisms through which export crops influence nutritional status may vary by commodity. This in turn might suggest that evaluation methods must have a large degree of flexibility and be adapted to each specific situation.

Coffee Production in Papua New Guinea

This example shows that two studies of the same area can lead to contradictory findings. Lambert [20] conducted a small survey in a coffee-growing area in New Guinea to determine whether cash cropping causes malnutrition. Food intake data were collected in 1975 for 13 households including 78 individuals. Data from this survey were compared to dietary intake data collected in 1956 when coffee production was first introduced into the area. The results showed that there was a 33% decline in food intake between the two periods, and that by 1975, the inhabitants had become even more heavily dependent on one food crop, the sweet potato.

Lambert [20] did not divide the dietary data by cash crop/noncash crop households. It would have been useful to separate the influence of cash crop production on household food intake from that of noncash crop. One of the weaknesses of this study is that the families surveyed in 1956 were not the same as those interviewed in 1975. Thus, we have no indication of whether or not families entering into coffee production were nutritionally better or worse off as a result of cash crop production. We only know that the aggregate community diet deteriorated between the two time periods. It is not clear whether this deterioration is associated with cash cropping or with some other external factor.

A second nutrition and growth study by Harvey and Heywood [16] was conducted in the same Simbu area of Papua New Guinea as the Lambert study [20]. The conclusions of the two studies are strikingly different. Harvey and Heywood [16], using a comparison of dietary data from 1956 (the baseline period for the Lambert study) and 1980/81, concluded that dietary intake had actually improved between the two time periods and that the contribution of sweet potato had decreased. They attribute much of this change to the better economic conditions that prevailed in the area as a result of cash crop production. One possible explanation for the diametrically opposite results of these two studies is a seasonal effect due to the timing of the Lambert study immediately after an important feast.

The three examples given above: Plan Chontalpa in Mexico, cash cropping in Kenya and coffee production in Papua New Guinea have in common the inability to conclude on the exact nature and causes of the nutritional differences observed. Because of unclear relationships between causes and effects, or contradictory findings for which there are no logical explanations, the conclusions remain tenuous and open to doubt.

Assessment of Technology for Work Alleviation in Burkina Faso

A factor which has been investigated as part of energy conservation techniques is the work load of project beneficiaries. Within a survey on human adaptation to low-energy intake in the Sahel regions [7, 10], the energy cost of drawing and fetching well water were measured. Women perform this work, which is very strenuous, in addition to their field work. The purpose of this study was to investigate to what extent the use of mechanical foot or hand pumps might alleviate women's work. Typical *daily* energy expenditures were calculated from two data sets.

One set was obtained from small groups of adult females who were carefully studied over 2- to 7-day periods during each season, the energy cost of their major activities were measured by indirect calorimetry, and their daily expenditures calculated. These energy costs were then applied to the second data set of Ancey [1] in which the daily pattern of activity of 900 adults and adolescents was recorded by interviewers over 1 year in five villages of Upper Volta. A total of 28,160 days of work were collected, with a classification in 41 activities.

In most villages, women and girls must walk to the closest well and carry 15–30 liters of water on their head several times a day. In the Sahel, water is drawn by hand using a receptacle and a rope to fill a jar. Our measurements were made to determine the amount of time and energy used to complete the task. These were compared to the energy cost of drawing water with a hand pump or a foot pump. This was done to assess the effect of several international programs to install pumps in villages.

All energy calculations were corrected for an average female adult body weight of 55 kg, irrespective of the percent of body fat. The traditional method of drawing water with a rope and a receptacle costs about five times the 'resting metabolic rate' per minute, which is the energy expenditure at complete rest. The energy cost per day of drawing water represents about 10% of the daily resting metabolic rate, or the energy equivalent of 40 g of cereals [9].

Participants were asked to pump water at their normal rate with appropriate mechanical pumps. The subjects pumped water at an average rate of 8.7 liters/min with the aid of the foot pump and 14.7 liters/min with the hand pump, that is 69% more per unit of time. In addition, the foot pump required 50% more energy per minute than the hand pump. The hand pump is therefore much more energy efficient than the foot pump. The depths of the wells were taken into account and correction factors used whenever necessary.

Another series of measurements showed that significantly less energy expenditure was required to draw 10 liters of water with a hand pump versus the traditional method using only a bucket and a rope. We concluded that the use of hand pumps appreciably improved the efficiency and speed with which women could draw water. The simple measure of human energy expenditure required to draw water using various methods permits quantitative comparison among them and could easily be used to assess other rural techniques. Projects have often ignored the extent to which interventions have affected the work load of the beneficiaries.

In another Burkina Faso study [10], the amount of time and energy required to prepare, husk and grind the staple cereals sorghum and millet was measured. This study as well as that of Ancey [1] indicate that an average of 1 h per adult women per day is spent preparing flour. This is equivalent to approximately 10% of the total daily energy expenditure spent preparing cereals, which is equal to 70 g of sorghum per woman per day, a substantial amount since daily consumption of grains is about 470 g/day. The four Sahelian countries (Senegal, Mali, Niger, and Burkina Faso) together have a population of 32 milion, of which it is estimated that 19 million depend on hand-husked and ground cereals. Although many rural women have access to a local hammer mill, the majority of them continue to hand grind for economic reasons. Every year, approximately 3.5 million metric tons of sorghum and millet are ground into flour by hand. This is the equivalent to a daily 8-hour pounding and grinding work shift by three-quarters of a million women.

Obviously, mechanical mills would reduce these strenuous chores. However, walking to and from the closest mill also requires time and energy which have to be included in the calculation. Observations made in villages in Burkina Faso indicate that in areas where the population is widely dispersed, the energy saved by using mills was minimal because of the distances that women had to walk. In addition, in order to pay for milling, women had to complete more handicraft work or procure cash from another source, imposing an additional financial burden on them. This example shows that the measurement of the impact of a new technology on work load can be measured, but that it needs to be placed in the context of a global perspective.

The Kirama Oya Basin, Sri Lanka, Development Scheme

In contrast to the previous examples of small-scale evaluations, this is an example of a much larger evaluation attempt. This detailed evaluation of an irrigation project in Sri Lanka was made to determine its effect on the nutritional status of the farming population [3]. For more than 6 years the Norwegian Development Agency (NORAD) funded the evaluation of a NORAD-supported Integrated Rural Development Program in the Hambantota District (HIRDEP). The goal was not only to evaluate the nutritional consequences of the project, but also to suggest additional ways in which the positive effects might be maximized. Field work was concentrated in the Kirama Oya Basin, a predominantly rice growing area, where project funds were spent to rehabilitate the irrigation system and to provide credit and insurance to small farmers.

The study included a large-scale nutrition survey made in August 1981 and subsequent monitoring of the nutritional situtation from August 1982 to August 1984. Data were collected including anthropometric measurements, dietary surveys, questionnaire interviews, and interviews with key informants. The researchers attempted to determine the magnitude and the causes of changes in the nutritional status of the beneficiaries of the Kirama Oya irrigated project. Comparisons were made with paddy farmers who received no water from Kirama Oya, and a group of poor households that had no access to paddy land. Diversity of ecological conditions between the study areas made the evaluation work complex.

The study team found that, in the Kirama region as a whole, from 1982 to 1984, general nutritional status improved significantly in the total sample (850 children) [3]. The prevalence of general malnutrition (both mild and severe) declined from 31 to 25%. Regionally, the nutritional status of preschool children improved in the northern part of the Kirama area, where the prevalence of general malnutrition declined from 39 to 22%. A similar improvement did not occur in the south, where there was no change in nutritional status. Positive nutritional and dietary changes took place in the lowest socioeconomic groups, while the medium and highest socioeconomic groups remained about the same. In 1984, the lowest income group seeemed to have caught up with the medium income group, both in terms of nutritional status and daily intake of staple foods.

In the region as a whole, the increase in agricultural production was only partly responsible for the general rise in income, which in turn could be traced to a high inflation rate. This was not only reflected in consumer food prices, but also in wholesale prices of agricultural commodities and agricultural wage rates. The improved nutritional status among children in the Kirama farmers' group could not be explained by a general decrease in the rate of infections or by improvements in the sanitary environment. In fact, data on disease patterns revealed that children of the Kirama farmers were slightly more likely to be sick than the children of the other paddy farmers' group not assisted by the project.

There were significant increases in paddy yields and in the percentages of the harvest that could be retained for home use by individuals in both project and nonproject farmers' group. However, the Kirama farmers harvested more than the control group. This was partly because of larger plot sizes and partly because of higher yields.

Table 1. Data collected in the surveys conducted in Gambia, Guatemala, Kenya and the Philippines

Variables	Method
Community-level variables	
Food prices	observe
Nonfood prices	observe
Population	record retrieval
Services available	observe
Household-level variables	
Socioeconomic information	recall
Income by source (agricultural, nonfarm, loans, other types)	recall
Income by individual earner	recall
Food expenditures	recall
Nonfood expenditures	recall
Energy consumption	recall
Water (source, distance)	recall
Sanitation (presence of latrine)	observe
Agricultural production (input by crop, production by crop)	recall
Storage of crops and agricultural inputs	recall
Labor input by crop and task, by household (adult and child), and by hired workers	recall
Women- and child-level variables	
Reproductive history	recall
Age	recall
Time allocation	recall
Weight, length, and weight for length	actual measurement
Preschooler energy intake[a]	recall by caretaker
Breastfeeding history and weaning practices	recall by mother
Morbidity patterns	recall
Mortality	recall

[a] Not available for all studies.
Source: E. Kennedy, J. von Braun, H. Bouis: Health and nutrition effects of the commercialization of agriculture: Evidence from the Gambia, Guatemala, Kenya, and the Philippines. Paper presented at Meeting of the Sub-Committee on Nutrition of the United Nations, Geneva 1988, p. 5.

Even though income data were similar for both groups of paddy farmers, a socioeconomic set of indicators for 1982 and 1984 showed that the Kirama farmers' material standard of living improved markedly. At the beginning of the evaluation, the socioeconomic indicators were actually lower for the Kirama farmers in 1982 than for other paddy farmers. During the 1982–1984 period the Kirama farmers 'caught up' with other farmers in terms of socioeconomic status.

This study in line with several others emphasizes the central role of women in child nutrition. The NORAD-supported nutritionists have tightly focussed on women as 'mediators' between the social and economic conditions outside the household and the nutritional situation of young children. Advances have been made in this study of the allocation of women's time and the impact of agricultural intervention such as cash cropping. However, the techniques to study time allocation as well as work loads and energy expenditures remain expensive and time consuming for large samples and more work is needed to develop these techniques.

A Comparative Study of Cash Cropping in Five Countries

This last series of examples shows also how the best designed evaluation methodologies have difficulties in identifying expected changes in nutritional status.

In a comparative study of cash crop and noncash crop households, von Braun et al. [29] found no significant differences in terms of growth (height, weight and weight for height) of children. They conducted five separate studies on commercialization of small holders of agriculture using nearly the same research protocol in the Gambia, Guatemala, Kenya, Rwanda and the Philippines. The variables measured in this remarkable series of studies are listed in table 1.

When heights and weights of children from traditional subsistence households were compared to those of children residing in households that planted commercial crops – irrigated paddy in the Gambia, horticultural crops for export in Guatemala, tea and potato schemes in Rwanda, and sugar cane in Kenya and the Philippines – there were no differences between the two groups. Although household income markedly increased in all five project areas following the adoption of commercial cropping, neither morbidity nor indicators of nutritional status showed a significant net improvement among preschoolers. Household mean food energy intake, as well as that for individual children, was higher in cash-cropping households when compared to traditional or subsistence households. However, because of poor environmental sanitation, the frequency of diarrhea and the prevalence of total illness were not reduced by increased income.

This example suggests that the nutritional impact of agricultural programs is extremely difficult to assess, even with well-designed research protocols. Alternatively, one could conclude that more sensitive and diversified indicators discussed below might be necessary. A standardized assessment procedure offers great advantages for cross-country comparative studies. However, each project may affect food and nutritional status in a rather specific manner. For example, diversity of food sources can be increased or decreased [12, 13], the stability of staple food supplies can be improved, and the availability of new foods can reduce the prevalence of common vitamin or mineral disorders without any measurable impact on children's growth (i.e., women iron deficiency anemia or vitamin A deficiency causing night blindness). In each of the above cases, a household food expenditure record, a dietary recall survey, or morbidity and anthropometry data collection might miss the key elements involved in change; diversity, stability, food security, and correction of specific nutritional deficiencies, which have no measurable effect on growth, but affects other physiological functions: work capacity, resistance to infection, duration for healing after a wound, or merely stamina and social relations.

Conclusion

The examples of project evaluations outlined in this chapter demonstrate some of the problems frequently encountered in nutritional impact evaluations. Often inadequate baseline data are used to assess changes, in many cases because evaluation is made late in the execution of the project rather than being incorporated early in the project design. In many studies the sample size is too small to detect statistically significant differences, many use indicators that are too restricted to capture changes that are likely to have occurred, and many ignore a possible impact on nonrecipients of the program. These examples demonstrate the need to broaden evaluation concepts and to increase the tools used to measure the impact of development projects on nutritional status.

Several points emerge on the importance of a broad view of the ways in which nutritional status could be affected by a particular type of development project, within a particular socioeconomic setting. For example, an irrigation project that provides water pumps to cash crop-producing landowners in an area with a high proportion of illiterate tenant farmers and landless laborers would be likely to have a very different impact on these various sectors of society, and through mechanisms that are not the same as those that could explain the impact of a project that provides high yielding varieties of staple crops to farmers in an area where land tenure is relatively equitable and there is a high rate of literacy. It is essential to be aware of the economic and social power relations in terms of access to resources such as land and credit that exist between recipients and nonrecipients in the country and of the potential market for the recipients' agricultural produce.

The design of an evaluation that is suited to the particular socioeconomic conditions of the project sites must therefore include several critical stages. A background study of the project should be made to determine the funding, its allocation, the stated and unstated objectives, and the intended beneficiaries. In addition, information on the socioeconomic setting has to be obtained, particularly in relation to the structure of land and water tenure, access to credit, other inputs and markets, dependency of the area on agriculture versus other income sources, the educational level of the population and the public health situation.

A picture of the lifestyle and work practices of the intended beneficiaries should be obtained, in particular allocation of tasks and resources within and outside the family at different seasons. Scenarios can then be envisaged of the effects the interventions are likely to have on the work patterns, production and income of the direct beneficiaries. The effect of these changes on their own nutrition and health situation, that of their dependents and on those who are not recipients of the program can then be considered how recipients may be affected by the consequent changes in food supply, food prices, land prices, environmental alterations, land availability, employment, etc.

The preparation of this scenario for evaluation is therefore an important process of imagination based on an understanding of the institutional and human limitations from a thorough background study. It is only within this type of broad view, fitted specifically to the local situation and its power structure, that decisions can sensibly be made about which sections of the population should be sampled for evaluation, which can serve as comparable controls, whether it is possible to design the evaluation to compare pre- and postintervention or only postintervention, the type of nutrition, health and socioeconomic information most likely to be useful, and the sample size required to provide reliable measure of differences. At this stage the appropriate tools can be chosen, from the array available, to indicate nutrition and health status and to understand why the intervention has or has not had a positive impact.

The examples used in this paper suggest that the range of techniques that can be used to assess the impact of agricultural projects on nutritional status can be very large. Examples of techniques that can be used where appropriate, to measure nutrition and health status, are anthropometry, morbidity, mortality, blood hemoglobin levels, biochemical indices of vitamin status. Examples of techniques used to explain these effects are measures of dietary intake diversity, questionnaires on weaning practices, parasite infestation, time allocation studies, measurement of energy expenditure for tasks specific to key sections of the population, particularly children and women.

The examples reviewed in this chapter demonstrate that quantifying nutritional changes resulting from intervention projects is both necessary and difficult. The difficulty arises because nutritional status can be assessed through various indicators and is affected by a large array of causal factors. However, the assessment is necessary to stimulate more effective interventions by identifying clearly which factors are responsible for which nutritional changes and how they could be enhanced. The theory that benefits of development project will 'trickle down' to the poorest individuals has frequently been proven wrong.

The history of attempts to include nutrition as a principal goal in development programs has been one of very limited success so far. In the early 1970s, nutritionists tried to influence development policies through food and nutrition planning at the national level [4]. In view of the difficulties of influencing government policy at the national level, with ministries of planning, there has been a change of emphasis towards incorporating nutritional objectives at the more manageable sectorial level and within agricultural development policies and programs. But even within this more limited scope a broad appropriate expertise is required.

Despite some promising advances, the infiltration of nutritional considerations into the sphere of agricultural development has been slow. Only a limited number of agricultural project documents from international development agencies or national ministries of agriculture include analyses that assess the effect of development strategies on consumption and nutrition. Many agricultural experts in governments and aid agencies do not yet regard nutrition as a serious field of interest [5]. They view nutrition as the domain of women and children, not as a specific objective of agricultural development. They are not familiar or comfortable dealing with nutritional issues even when they recognize it as important and concentrate on objectives considered to be of higher priority: production, export, economic considerations. However, integrating nutritional considerations into an agricultural agenda remains critically important.

As we demonstrated, one of the reasons that nutritionists have had little success in this area is that they have not adequately developed the combination of an ability to analyze the social and economic determinants of nutrition with the technical tools required to monitor the nutritional and health-related impacts of agricultural interventions. However, this chapter shows that methodologies and specific parameters to measure nutritional impact in a comprehensive manner are now emerging, but require more attention from the nutrition community. A practical manual may be required to speed this progress in which both methods to analyze specific socioeconomic relationships at the project site and the technical methods for measuring impact are described along with suggestions for deciding on which of the array of techniques would be appropriate.

Efforts to identify sturdy portable equipment for field studies of that nature have been initiated [15]. Unfortunately, many of the techniques for nutritional evaluation such as quantitative food intake are long and tedious, or quite imprecise. Methods for rapid appraisal of nutritional situations need to be developed by nutritionists to provide the critical information needed by agronomists and planners sympathetic to their objectives, and in so doing, grasp unique opportunities to assist aid agencies in eradicating or at least reducing severe malnutrition by appropriate agricultural policies and relevant projects.

References

1   Ancey, G.: Facteurs et systèmes de production dans la société Mossi d'aujourd'hui (Office de la Recherche Scientifique et Technique d'Outre-Mer, Ouagadougou 1974).
2   Barrett, M.; Lassiter, S.; Wilcock, D.; Baker, D.; Crawford, E.: Animal traction in Eastern Upper Volta: A technical, economic and institutional analysis. MSU International Development Paper No. 4, (Department of Economics, Michigan State University, East Lansing 1982).
3   Barth, E.W.: Introducing nutritional considerations into rural development programs with focus on agriculture. Report No. 3. Nutritional Evaluation of the Kirama

Oya Basin Development Scheme in Hambantota, Sri Lanka (Institute for Nutrition Research, Oslo 1986).

4   Berg, A.: The Nutrition Factor (Brookings Institute, Washington 1973).

5   Berg, A.; Austin, J.: Nutrition policies and programmes: A decade of redirection. Food Policy 9: 304–312 (1984).

6   Bleiberg, F.M.; Brun, T.A.; Goihman, S.; Lippman, D.: Food intake and energy expenditure of male and female farmers from Upper Volta. Br. J. Nutr. 45: 505–515 (1981).

7   Bleiberg, F.M.; Brun, T.A.; Goihman, S.; Gouba, E.: Duration of activities and energy expenditure of female farmers in dry and rainy seasons in Upper Volta. Br. J. Nutr. 43: 71–82 (1980).

8   Brun, T.A.: Intégration de considérations nutritionnelles dans les programmes de développement rural, Haïti. Expérimentation de la méthodologie et proposition de projets pour renforcer l'impact alimentaire des projets de développement rural. TCP/HAI/0107 (FAO, Rome 1982).

9   Brun, T.A.: Coût énergétique comparé du puisage traditionnel de l'eau, du pompage manuel et à pied au Burkina. Coll. Inst. Natl. Santé Rech. Méd. 136: 285–292 (1986).

10   Brun, T.A.; Bleiberg, F.M.; Bonny, S.; Ancey, G.: Alimentation et dépense énergétique du paysan Mossi. Environnement Africain, ENDA-UNICEF; Special issue on children and adolescents in Sudanian and Sahelian Environments, Dakar, Senegal, Nos 14–16, vol. IV, pp. 2–4 (1980).

11   Cernea, M.M.: Measuring project impact: Monitoring and evaluation in the PIDER Rural Development Project, Mexico. World Bank Staff Working Paper No. 332 (World Bank, Washington 1979).

12   Dewey, K.G.: Agricultural development, diet and nutrition. Ecol. Food Nutr. 8: 265–273 (1979).

13   Dewey, K.G.: Nutritional consequence of the transformation from subsistence to commercial agriculture in Tabasco, Mexico. Human Ecol. 9: 151–186 (1981).

14   Fitchet, D: Staff appraisal report Puno Rural Development Project-Peru, Report No. 2736-PE (World Bank, Washington 1980).

15   Geissler, C.; Saravanabavandan, P.; Croor, S.: Field equipment for nutrition and health studies (Kings College, University of London, 1988).

16   Harvey, P.; Heywood, P.: Twenty-five years of dietary change in Simbu Province, Papua New Guinea. Ecol. Food Nutr. 13: 27–35 (1983).

17   Hernandez, M.; Hidalgo, C.P.: Effect of economic growth in nutrition in a typical community. Ecol. Food Nutr. 3: 283–391 (1974).

18   Hitchings, J.: Agricultural determinants of nutritional status among Kenyan children with model of anthropometric and growth indicators; PhD diss. Stanford University, Palo Alto (1982).

19   Kennedy, E.T.; Cogill, B.: Income and Nutritional Effects of the Commercialization of Agriculture in Southwestern Kenya. Research Report 67 (International Food Policy Research Institute, Washington 1987).

20   Lambert, J.N.: Does cash cropping cause malnutrition? (National Planning Office, Port Moresby, Papua New Guinea 1978).

21   Lele, U.: The Design of Rural Development: Lessons from Africa (Johns Hopkins University Press, Baltimore 1975).

22   Lev, L.: The effect of cash cropping on food consumption adequacy among the Meru of Northern Tanzania. Working Paper No. 21 (Michigan State University, East Lansing 1981).

23   Lunven, P.: The nutritional consequences of agricultural and rural development projects. Food Nutr. Bull. *4:* (1982).

24   Palmer, I.: The New Rice in Asia: Conclusions from Four Country Studies (United Nations Research Institute for Social Development, Geneva 1976).

25   Popkin, B.M.; Solon, F.S.; Fernandez, T.L.; Latham, M.C.: Benefit-cost analysis in the nutrition area. A project in the Philippines. Soc. Sci. Med. *14C:* 207–216 (1980).

26   Solon, F.; Fernandez, T.L.; Latham, M.C.; Popkin, B.M.: An evaluation of strategies to control vitamin A deficiency in the Philippines. Am. J. Clin. Nutr. *32:* 1445–1453 (1979).

27   Sornmani, S.; Schelp, F.P.; Sesth, V.; Pongpaew, P.; Sritabutra, P.; Supawan, V.; Vudhivai, N.; Egormaiphul, S.; Harinasuta, C.: An investigation of the health and nutritional status of the population in the Nam Pong Water Resource Development Project, Northeast Thailand. Am. Trop. Med. Parasitol *75:* 335–346 (1981).

28   United Nations University: Methods for the Evaluation of the Impact of Food and Nutrition Programmes. Food Nutr. Bull., Suppl. 8 (The United Nations University, Tokyo 1984).

29   Von Braun, J.; Kennedy,E.; Bouis, H.: Commercialization of Smallholder Agriculture: A Comparative Analysis of the Effects on Household Level, Food, Security and Nutrition and Implications for Policy. Final Report submitted to SLD, PPC, Washington (1988).

30   World Bank: Rural Development Projects: A Retrospective View of Bank Experience in Sub-Saharan Africa. Report No. 2242 (World Bank, Washington 1978).

31   World Bank: Nutritional Consequences of Agricultural Projects: Conceptual Relationships and Assessment Approaches. World Bank Staff Working Paper No. 456 (World Bank, Washington 1981).

T.A. Brun, PhD, Division of Nutritional Science, Cornell University, Ithaca, NY 14853 (USA)

Simopoulos AP (ed): Impacts on Nutrition and Health.
World Rev Nutr Diet. Basel, Karger, 1991, vol 65, pp 124–162

The Nutrition and
Health Impact of Cash Cropping in West Africa:
A Historical Perspective

Thierry A. Brun[1]

Institut Agronomique Méditerranéen, Centre International des Hautes Etudes
Méditerranéennes, Montpellier and Institut National de la Santé et de la
Recherche Médicale Paris, France

Contents

[1] I want to express my deepest gratitude to Bonnie Sterling, Tammy Benjamin and
Francine Whitted for typing and editing the manuscript and to Catherine Geissler, Simon
Maxwell, Eileen Kennedy, and Mike Pitzrick for assistance in reviewing the draft of this
paper and suggesting corrections.

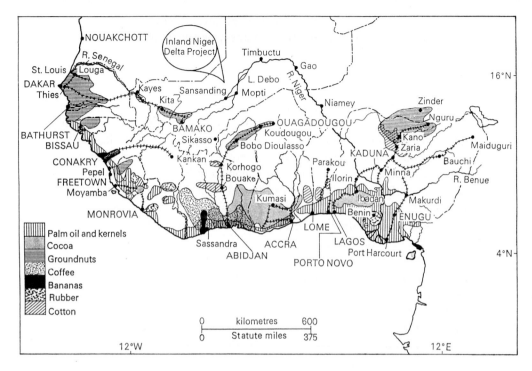

Fig. 1. Main areas of export crop production in the 1960s [data from 15].

Introduction

In half a century, cash cropping, or the production of crops primarily for sale to European traders, has spread over thousands of hectares in West Africa (fig. 1). It now occupies the most fertile and the best irrigated lands. Cash cropping, subsistence agriculture and human nutrition have seldom been studied together in order to clarify their interrelationship. Like all scientific questions which cut across disciplines, the study of the impact of cash cropping on nutrition is both difficult and somewhat frustrating. Although one feels that it must have a considerable influence on food production, consumption and therefore nutritional status of populations, there is very little evidence of such clear relationship in the literature [9, 10, 13, 18, 22, 31].

Ecological conditions, population density, and social organization vary considerably from region to region in West Africa and the history of the expansion of each cash crop is quite often different from one to the other. Therefore, it is not possible to make broad generalizations. We shall rather select a few significant examples which illustrate indirectly the impact of cash cropping on food consumption and nutritional status in some countries.

Some authors have attempted to distinguish the effects of export cropping from those of colonial domination. Cash cropping cannot be separated, in our opinion, from the whole context of precolonial trade, colonial domination from the beginning of the century until 1960, and neocolonial dependency after 1960. Similarly, food consumption and nutritional status are only one facet of the quality of life and we must keep in mind a global view of the social impact of commercial agriculture if we want to understand how food production and consumption have evolved over time in rural areas of West Africa.

We shall see how the need for specific tropical products led to colonial domination of African chiefdoms and later to significant investments in West Africa. This is documented by reviewing the interpretations of economic historians on the effects of the colonial era in shaping the present agricultural situation in West Africa. The example of the Office du Niger, located in Mali, will be used. The relationship between export cropping, French administration, and local social structures appear clearly in examples from the Ivory Coast and Burkina Faso (Upper Volta until 1984).

We shall examine the impact of cash cropping on human resources: the institution of forced labor, the changes which occurred in the role of women, and how the criteria of power and wealth were profoundly modified. Cash cropping led to a new type of agriculture which has been termed 'mining' agriculture because it resulted in extensive soil deterioration. The lack of innovation in export cropping in the Sahel countries and the loss of prestige of traditional food crops will also be illustrated. Two further chapters will document the most significant impact of cash cropping which has occurred through rapid monetarization. Taxes imposed by colonial powers and a variety of financial pressures on peasants have limited capital accumulation among producers and therefore prevented a gradual increase in productivity. The last chapters deal more specifically with consumption patterns and nutritional status as they relate to cash crop earnings.

In conclusion, we shall present alternative development strategies and suggest that export cropping is more likely to have a positive economic (and consequently nutritional) impact when producers are organized in such a way as to control in part the marketing of their production.

Colonization and Cash Cropping

There are varying viewpoints on the impact of the colonial era in shaping the present economical, agricultural and food supply situation in West Africa. Historians such as Hopkins [15] believed colonialism had only a limited effect, and in his 'Economic History of West Africa' he states:

> There are sound reasons for thinking that colonial rule itself had a less dramatic and a less pervasive economic impact than was once supposed. Little more than half a century elapsed between the end of the partition of West Africa and the beginning of independence. The first fifteen years of this period were devoted to pacifying recalcitrant peoples, the last fifteen years were spent trying to cope with African nationalism, and the intervening years provide plenty of evidence of the superficiality and impermanence of colonial rule, even though this was the time when the rulers themselves believed that their paternal control would remain unchallenged for several centuries.

Other authors have credited colonial domination with most of the social and economic progress made by West African countries since the turn of the century. They specifically cite the development of the export sector and the establishment of connections with the modern (international) market economy as positive contributions to existing West African economies. However, when the 1973 famine occurred in the Sahel countries, colonial heritage and in particular groundnut and cotton cultivation were blamed for deteriorating soils, distracting scare resources from cereal production and providing an exaggerated income to an urban minority to the detriment of the rural masses.

Are commercial farming and export cropping a healthy base for economic development, or have they been the instruments of exploitation, environmental destruction and the cause of recent food shortages and massive imports in West Africa? In view of the severity of the nutritional problems of the Sahel countries and the magnitude of food imports and food aid in West Africa, a study of the past, present and future role of cash cropping is of utmost importance.

An evaluation of the nature of the impact of the colonial era requires a clarification of the philosophy that underlined the colonial presence in West Africa. In the late 30s the French government already had control of a vast empire, extending over 11 million km^2 from the Caribbean to Indochina, and affecting more than 100 million people. However, France's largest possessions were in Africa. The following example selected from

French West Africa illustrates several aspects of the social impact of commercial cotton cultivation as it was conceived and implemented by French investors and French administration.

The Office du Niger: Cotton Cultivation in West Africa

Between 1905 and 1910, the French textile industry had to import 75% of its raw cotton from the USA. The US textile industry was expanding rapidly and processing an increasing percentage of its own cotton production; this amount increased from one third in 1900 to one half in 1913. In France, the whole cotton industry, which employed over 250,000 workers, was threatened by the forthcoming shortages of raw cotton and the strong position of the US textile industry [36]. This situation was further aggravated by World War I as the reduction in maritime traffic limited the opportunity to import raw cotton to Europe. From 1916 to 1924, both world production and consumption stagnated. Prices, however, soared from 73 to 276 francs in New York for 50 kg of 'cotton middling', and from 78 to 408 francs in Le Havre (the largest market for raw cotton in France).

In 1903, 'L'Association Cotonnière Coloniale' (ACC) had been created by the 'Syndicat Général de l'Industrie Cotonnière Française' to encourage cotton production overseas. During the 15 years which followed, a number of colonial associations, companies, and committees carried on campaigns which made colonization of Africa a national duty and a major issue in Parliament, government and financial circles. 'France's salvation will come from our colonies' was the new slogan. The exploitation of our tropical empire became a patriotic venture [36].

It is surprising that such high expectations could have been sustained so long when one considers the disappointing results of cotton cultivation in French Sudan from 1904 to 1913. The cost of production of nonirrigated new varieties of American cotton in Sudan was twice the price of US imported cotton in Le Havre.

For the Sudanese farmers, cotton production required more work than tradionally grown millet and was more susceptible to pests and parasites than millet. Cotton growing had a profit margin of 15 francs/hectare whereas millet would leave a profit of 100–150 francs/hectare. Peasants were so upset by the low prices paid to them by the ACC for cotton that they preferred to store their harvest from October to April and sell it, at a higher price, to nomadic tribes. During the same period, Egyptian varieties of irrigated cotton were tested in Senegal. The low yields made it unreasonable for the native farmers to continue to grow cotton. Therefore, the Governor-General Clozel, in a correspondence dated April 24, 1912, instructed district commissioners[2] to make it mandatory for natives to plant cotton [36]. French district commissioners were also instructed to make sure that cotton was sold directly to ACC, which continued to buy cotton at a lower price than farmers could sell it on the market.

It is in this context that the civil engineer Belime was commissioned in 1919–1920 to explore the possibility of growing irrigated cotton on a large scale between Bamako, in Southwest Mali, and Lake Debo, North of Mopti. Belime, who had studied the British irrigation techniques in India, wrote a detailed report demonstrating that constructing three irrigation networks in Segou, Nyamina and Sansanding would open to cultivation 1.3 million hectares. One third of this acreage could be dedicated to cotton cultivation and produce enough for the entire French textile industry. Belime estimated that over 1 million native peasants would be needed to cultivate such extensive acreage of cotton. In 1919, French Sudan had a population estimated at 3 million inhabitants. The project area included only half a million people of which 300,000 were farmers, and the lack of manpower to cultivate such extensive acreage of cotton was a major obstacle.

The Minister of Colonies, Albert Sarraut, also believed that human manpower was the critical factor:

Our policy towards natives must give higher priority to education and medical care because the working potential (of the population) is the key to the exploitation of the colonies (Sarraut, 1923; in Schreyer [36]).

Despite this awareness, and the concern expressed by representatives for the well-being of the native population of West Africa, it was not long before reports were circulated which documented the use of brutal force in the transplantation of populations to conduct forced labor on railways, roads and other works of public interest. The food situation in the region had not improved significantly since the famine of 1913–1914, which claimed thousands of lives in the Sahel regions. In 1924, another famine occurred in the districts of Segou, Issa-Ber and Timbuktu. Governor-General Darde was concerned by the grain shortage and demanded that rice should also be grown on the newly irrigated lands.

---

[2] In French 'Commandant de Cercle'.

In 1920, Hirsh led a group of major French banks to invest in the 'Compagnie de Culture Cotonnière du Niger' (CCCN). This consortium obtained immediately a loan of 280 million francs from the State. The CCCN had a concession of 2,000 hectares in the region of Dire, in Northeast Mali. However, its relationship to peasants deteriorated to the point that many fled home. Their wages were significantly lower than in Kayes and Bamako and the company would withold part of their pay, allegedly as 'savings', as a measure to force them to stay. Hygiene and medical care were appalling. Although the Governor-General Jules Carde condemned its methods in 1924, the CCCN continued unchanged and still received state financial support, thanks to its banking lobby in Paris.

In the meantime, Belime and his supporters had convinced the Parisian circles that the Niger Inner Delta was comparable to the Nile valley [36]. The construction of the dam and canals of Sotuba, which was initiated in 1925, was entrusted to the 'Service Temporaire des Irrigations du Niger' (STIN) under the direction of Lieutenant-Colonel Doizelet. He used forced labor. Food, nutrition and hygiene were appalling during the first 2 years, and the number of deaths, work accidents and fugitives was quite high. During the first year, out of 1,850 forced laborers over 100 died, an equal number fled and over 200 were injured and disabled. The following year, out of 2,850 laborers, 13% died, 24% fled and 32% were disabled. During the third year immunization and an improvement of the basic diet significantly reduced the death toll [36].

Belime managed to find financial support and to survive several budget crises, and in 1932, the projet became a state enterprise under the name of 'Office du Niger'. However, out of the 960,000 hectares of irrigated land promised in 1924, only 13,000 were actually irrigated in 1929. Total production of cotton did not exceed 422 tons (100,000 tons had been planned) and rice production was hardly 6,200 tons. All this for the exorbitant cost of 12 billion francs.

A major reason for this failure was that most of the peasants had been forced to settle and work on the project. As local farmers from Segou refused to move from their villages to the irrigated areas, several campaigns and site visits were organized to convince the chief of the Mossi, and the Moro-Naba in Upper Volta to find 'volunteers' to work in Mali. A large operation of recruiting was organized in the Ouahigouya, Tougan and Koutiala regions in 1942. Many peasants knew that the Office du Niger was similar to a 'work camp'. In order to escape, young men migrated by the thousands from Upper Volta to the Ivory Coast. In their villages of origin, the elders were complaining bitterly that they had lost either to Mali or the Ivory Coast work force on which they depended to produce millet and sorghum for their survival. Village leaders would designate those they wanted to punish as volunteers to work in Mali. Those who were forced to settle in the Office du Niger complained of the low price of cotton, the absence of women to marry and the administrative obstacle to their return home even for family events.

The administration had forbidden women to grow vegetables as this would distract them from working on cotton cultivation. Hygiene, nutrition and medical attention were so poor that between 1934 and 1944 the number of deaths (6,570 individuals) was almost as high as the number of births (6,959 babies) [36].

In 1944, 1,000 Bambara settlers asked to leave the irrigation project and in 1945, out of 23,500 dwellers, over 5,500 actually left to return home. Towards the end of World War II, the 'Ministre des Colonies' asked the Governor-General Reste to conduct an appraisal mission of the situation in the Office du Niger, in view of a general reorganization. In addition to numerous technical errors, the mission found that the social situation was distressful and that the absence of humanitarian concern for the dignity and participation of the peasants was a major factor in the failure and the exorbitant cost of the whole project.

There are several lessons to be learned from this example. The genuine need for raw material, in this instance cotton, led major banking institutions to mislead the French public and manipulate politicians to their advantage. Private investors in French West Africa obtained generous loans and grants, and were allowed access to navy and army facilities to transport, build and organize their trade to and from Africa. Thus, considerable sums of money from taxpayers were dedicated to the creation of profitable private enterprises under the banner of national access to primary products needed by the French textile industry.

Unilever: The Presence of Multinationals in West Africa

Cash cropping from West Africa was the major source of capital for multinationals such as Unilever. When William H. Lever felt the need for more oils and fats to expand its production of soap, he sent out his own explorers to Africa [33] and between 1910 and 1920 he bought several small companies from West Africa, including the Niger Company in 1920. Lever also merged with a number of competitors and in 1929 he merged with a Dutch rival and created the monopoly Unilever. By the end of the colonial period, Unilever was a world force selling traditional soaps, detergents, margarine, cooking oil, canned foods, candles, glycerine, oil cake and toilet preparations [33].

According to the information division of the Unilever House in London itself, the company's largest source of profits was Africa. These profits were obtained both by purchasing their oils and fats from Africa and, in turn, selling 'all kinds of goods' to African peasants. The African branch of Unilever, the United Africa Company (UAC), allowed the manufacturing side of Unilever to have control over a guaranteed source of raw materials [33]. As the French 'compagnies de traite', Unilever decided that they should also invest in retail distribution. Therefore, Unilever purchased chains of grocery stores.

West Africa was soon invaded by hoards of Lebanese shopkeepers who would act as intermediaries for European traders. The same French family enterprises, which from Bordeaux or Nantes accumulated a fortune on slave trade in the 18th century, continued in the 19th century in the form of legal trade with West Africa. Powerful consortia such as the 'Société Commerciale de l'Ouest Africain' (SCOA) had the backing of major French banks. Unilever had a subsidiary, NOSOCO, which would buy palm oil and groundnuts directly from the producers. In this way, cash cropping was directly connected to the supply of groceries and household goods in West Africa. Peasants would obtain loans until the next harvest from their usual suppliers of basic commodities: rice, salt, sugar, cooking oil, fabric, etc. and, in turn, the retailers would obtain loans from leading foreign trading firms. The cash paid at the harvest was meticulously drained back by the same trading companies from Europe.

Human Resources and Cash Cropping

Export cropping needed labor to produce the desired harvest but also to transport the harvest to the coast. This was especially apparent in the dense forest region of the Ivory Coast. The absence of draft animals led the French administration to recruit by force thousands of natives to transport on their heads loads averaging 50–55 lbs for distances in excess of 100 miles.

In the mid-60s, Meillassoux [24] conducted an extensive historical study on the Gourou territory of the Ivory Coast. At the end of the 19th century, this area was peopled by various native tribes. The Gourous themselves were a self-sufficient ethnic group who primarily hunted. They were also able to harvest a plentiful supply of cola nuts, highly valued as an item of trade by other groups further north. According to Meillassoux, the economic goals of colonization at the beginning of the century were straightforward and openly acknowledged: the exploitation of ivory and rubber without any concern for the welfare of the local population. His account clearly documents the severity of the impact of colonization on social organizations, trade and social values.

The French were convinced that Gourou country was rich in ivory and rubber. The territory was first included in a military 'cercle' in 1902. A series of violent incidents broke out between the Gourous and native traders, and the French army closed the area to the traders. The Gourou protested, and in 1906, the following conditions were mandated by the French to reinstate normal trade [24]: (a) installation of whites (military) throughout the territory; (b) free traffic in trade; (c) settlement of all conflicts and disputes by the legal system of the whites; (d) institution of a tax to be paid to the administration; (e) transportation of goods by natives (with pay); (f) compulsory work for the maintenance of roads. These conditions, in effect, put the territory under colonial rule.

The Gourou did not accept French military occupation, and refused to pay taxes, to supply men to carry loads for long distances or to participate in the construction of roads, etc. Their resistance lasted more than 8 years. During this time, French troops destroyed villages, burnt granaries, and killed thousands of villagers. Statistics from January to October 1912 are revealing: the French occupation troops lost 10 black soldiers and 44 were injured; the Gourous lost 1,400 men, women and children. Out of 115 documented villages, 53 had been burnt during the French 'conquest' [24]. In 1914, the Gourou and other tribes of the area were finally forced to disarm and submit. They were then considered by the French to fall under existing French West Africa colonial laws. By a 1901 decree, all men, women and adolescents aged 10 years or more had to pay a tax (originally set for the Ivory Coast at 2.5 francs/year). The French also relocated the Gourou into specified areas in order to facilitate administration of the region, and to make the population more accessible to the work to be done.

During this period, it was the army's responsibility to open roads and transport products to the coast, and consequently to conscript native workers. A report dated 1917 states that a column of 9,500 'porteurs' transported 235 tons of rice, rubber, cotton, corn, palm oil, seeds, etc. In actuality, the Gourous never stopped resisting. A number of them refused to collect rubber and pay taxes. Whole villages were found empty and abandoned when the army tried to recruit 'volunteers'. Villagers attempted to escape to the forest, and the army followed, destroying their encampments.

In 1924, the deterioration of the situation led to the appointment of Colonial Inspector Merat. He reported that, 'Forced transportation was imposing more strenuous work on peasants than they were prepared to tolerate'. It varied from 12 to 80 days per adult per year. He recommended that 'compulsory work' be reduced. Instead, the French administration decided to institute a system of forced labor which lasted from 1925 to 1946.

European investors were increasingly involved with agricultural production and foresting in the territory and needed a larger and larger work force. Recruitment of workers for private concerns already existed, whereby local chiefs contracted to supply men to foreign-owned plantations and lumber camps. By a 1925 decree, contractual work agreements between private concerns and individual Gourous were established. These agreements were supposedly voluntary, but in actuality the Gourous were not informed of this difference from other public work consignments. In effect, the army and the administration became the suppliers of cheap labor to private coffee and cocoa growers. A number of reports revealed the conditions of workers: housed in filthy, tiny shelters, receiving insufficient food and inadequate clothing, with almost no medical assistance for those who were sick. Several medical inspections showed that workers were lean, underfed, with marks of beatings that had not received treatment. Average weights varied between 50 and 60 kg for men aged 17–40. Some were even less than 45 kg [24]. A considerable number of laborers ran away from the planations. Meillassoux [24] reviewed a number of reports where the percentage of fugitives varied from 10 to 62%. In order to reduce the number, the French administration made the fugitive's village of origin responsible for him. The village chief had to immediately designate someone to replace the individual who ran away. Villages were also forced to replace workers who were sick or injured.

Forced labor was responsible for thousands of deaths in Africa. Between May and June 1892, out of the 4,500 men who worked on the construction of the Congo-Ocean railroad (from Matadi to Stanley-Pool), 900 (20%) died as the railway extended only 90 km, an average of 10 lives lost per kilometer. Forced labor took men from their villages without consideration for the shortage of labor at the time of planting or weeding.

Whole villages with a large number of women and children were left without the necessary assistance and protection of a sufficient number of adult men. Moreover, it created a constant fear of being dragged away for so-called 'public' works. 'Administration' became the symbol of ruthless exploitation, unfair punishment and unkept promises, and a general distrust of any administrative rule developed. At any one time, only 5% or less of the Gourou adult males were engaged in forced labor in the construction of roads and railroads or as farm workers on plantations. But in order to obtain a constant rotation and renewal of this manpower, it was necessary to subjugate the entire population of 76,000 individuals. Needless to say, forced laborers were not motivated, and productivity and work efficiency was low. The fact that many ran away further contributed to this inefficiency.

The institution of forced labor increased civil unrest, crime rate and repression by the colonial administration. Colonizers used and abused human resources as they did the land and demonstrated little concern for the welfare of the stock of native manpower. It was indeed a very destructive system. The cost of manpower was very low for plantations and local foreign enterprises. The whole colonial infrastructure was financed by European taxpayers. When forced labor was abolished in 1946, and the administration no longer supplied any cheap laborers to plantations, most owners were unable to pay for the work they required and consequently foreign investment could not be maintained. In the Ivory Coast, from the early 50s onward, the cultivation of coffee and cocoa was taken over almost exclusively by native growers.

Taxation, Trade, and Groundnut Expansion

Some have argued that there were positive compensations to those severe conditions: wages were paid to workers, generating economic development. As a matter of fact, wages were paid, but they were ridiculously low. From 1927 to 1938 wages remained unchanged: 2 francs/day in the plantation and 2.5 francs in the forest lumber exploitation sites. In 1938, it was increased by 0.50 francs and in 1944 it reached respectively 3.50 and 4 francs. Adolescents aged 14–17 were paid 2.5 francs/day. By 1940, in a number of districts those wages were sometimes not sufficient to cover the various taxes and fees to which the population was subject. Taxes increased at a much faster rate than wages and in 1943, each person above

10 years of age had to pay 85 francs, the equivalent of a month and a half of work. To pay taxes alone, the head of the household with many dependents had to work several months.

In French colonies, for several centuries, trade with natives from tropical countries was called 'traite'. It referred, according to the dictionary Littré, to 'any trade or exchange of goods with savages'. Peasants would take their groundnut harvest to traders[3] who would offer in turn rice, millet, sugar, edible oil, kerosene, alcohol, fabric, bicycles and watches. Although money was used, this type of trade was similar to bartering. Money was spent almost entirely for immediate purchases and payment of outstanding loans. The 'traitants' would loan money at usurious rates to their groundnut or cotton suppliers. Interest rates varied between 100 and 250% a year in Sahel countries [17]. Recent studies show that 80–90% of the loans are not spent on agriculture. The loans are guaranteed by the next cash crop harvest. In general the peasants sell their next harvest at a much lower price than they could obtain later.

The impact of the extension of groundnut cultivation on social and economic life has been studied extensively by Raynaut [32] in the region of Maradi in Niger. He shows conclusively that food shortages and famines, which have been more frequent in this region since the mid-60s, result from several factors linked to the circulation of cash. When taxation was first imposed, most peasants were forced to cultivate either cotton or groundnut in order to pay their taxes and that of their family. Then, gradually, as a number of goods and commercial foods became commonly used there has been an increasing pressure on heads of extended families to devote a larger and larger fraction of their time and land to groundnut cultivation. One striking feature of cash income, in Raynaut's view, is the speed at which it is recycled. As soon as the groundnut harvest has been sold, the head of the traditional household faces a number of urgent expenses: taxes to the government, debts to various traders, ceremonies, presents and a number of other social obligations. Almost nothing is ever saved for delayed consumption and even less kept for productive investments.

Already in 1954, the expansion of groundnut in areas traditionally dedicated to millet and sorghum was critical. The risks of food shortages became such, that the Governor of Niger instructed all 'Commandants de Cercle' in this manner:

---

[3] Traders responsible for the collection of groundnut and other cash crops were called 'traitants'.

Groundnut cultivation has now reached a level which should, under no circumstances, be exceeded. Despite the advantageous price offered to the producer, the extension (of groundnut) at the expense of food crops appears dangerous. You will make sure that not a single hectare of millet or other food crop should be distracted by peasants to the benefit of groundnut cultivation and I ask you to invite all our 'Chefs de circonscription' not to spare any effort in the coming months to fight against this tendency (Archives du Président de la République, Niamey; in Raynaut [32]).

The legitimate concern of this French governor would not have led to such measures, had not the deterioration of the food situation been amply documented. However, this did not stop groundnut expansion and from 26,000 tons in the Cercle of Maradi in 1954 it extended threefold and reached 75,000 tons in 1966 (yield/hectare did not increase). Thanks to the selection of varieties with a shorter cycle, groundnut was able to compete with millet in areas where this last crop was previously unchallenged. Millet in turn was pushed northward where rainfall was lower, the risk of drought higher and yield inevitably lower.

New Sets of Values with Cash Economy

The accelerated development of groundnut cultivation between 1920 and 1961 gradually deteriorated the prestige of millet and sorghum; beer, wine and other alcoholic beverages could replace the fermented sorghum beer. In the eyes of farmers, millet and sorghum were no longer essential crops. Cash and therefore cash-generating crops became indispensable to village leaders and heads of households to pay taxes, to buy clothes, tools, bicycles, watches, radios, cooking utensils, meat, spices, etc.

As the market economy expanded, men were under increasing financial pressure. This also generated tensions among the traditional extended African family. Sons would no longer work for their father. They preferred to obtain a separate piece of land to cultivate or to migrate to plantations or urban centers. The migration caused by cash cropping expansion after World War II also contributed to social disruption and poverty in the Sahel countries. In the late 50s, it was estimated that at least 100,000 would migrate every year from Upper Volta, Dahomey and Togo to the Ivory Coast. In turn, from the Ivory Coast thousands would migrate to Ghana [1]. In 1965, it was estimated that in the Ivory Coast, out of a total population of 3.8 million, 1 million were originally from other regions: 0.5 million from Upper Volta, 200,000 from Mali and 200,000 from Guinea [1].

The intensity of the need for 'cash' was, according to Raynaut [32], the leading factor of groundnut expansion, migration and urbanization: cities meant potential jobs and wages. In addition, governments have increased progressively taxes levied from peasants. In 1952, a peasant had to sell 24 kg of shelled groundnut to pay the tax for 1 person. In 1963, he had to sell 40 kg, and 1970 he had to sell 70 kg. In the meantime, groundnut prices have increased from 16 francs CFA/kg in 1952 to 24 francs CFA in 1963 and declined to 21 francs CFA in 1970.

Another feature of cash cropping expansion has been the introduction of inappropriate technologies. Even the animal-drawn plough which has been so widely recommended is not necessarily the answer. There is evidence that the technical advantages of the type of plough commercialized by the French, then by the national agricultural extension departments, have been grossly exaggerated. In most circumstances, given the type of constraints faced by peasants, uncertainty of the rainfall and the lack of spare parts and repair shops, it is unwise for an isolated farmer to invest in an animal-drawn plough. Only if the same plough is shared by several farm units, can its use by justified on economic grounds.

Any innovation and any investment represents a considerable risk for the peasant, since he is totally unable to predict his harvest. Buying a draft animal might force him to sell part of his possessions, or necessitate loans to buy millet essential to survival. If he is forced to sell land that he owns and cultivates, he can be pushed into a self-perpetuating spiral of impoverishment. This often led to misunderstandings and conflicts between extension workers and peasants. Most extension workers were trained to maximize yields per hectare as generally done in Europe. For peasants with limited funds to invest in expensive groundnut seed, the limiting factor is often the quantity of seed or the quantity of physical labor, not the land acreage.

The lack of innovation and the backwardness of present cultivation techniques in the Sahel can be explained in large part by the poor adaptation of most of the techniques recommended by extension services. For example, fertilizers have proven difficult to use where rainfall is so unpredictable. As is well known, fertilizers are useless when rain is insufficient, and can be a major expense for the farmer.

In West Africa there have been few innovations in the production of groundnut. The adoption of new varieties and the use of pesticides were the most important achievements. Mechanization did not progress as had been predicted and yield remained low. Had it not been for the constant support and sometime constraints of colonial rule, groundnut and cotton cultivations would not have reached their present extension. In many instances, their production was less profitable than sorghum and millet cultivation.

In Maradi, in 1974, Raynaut [32] shows conclusively that if the time spent by the peasants is valued at the cost of hired labor it does not pay to cultivate groundnut. Groundnut requires a minimum of 60 days and more frequently 100 days/hectare at 125–190 francs CFA/day. Yields are usually close to 700 kg providing an income of 10,500 francs CFA which is therefore lower than the value of the farmer's work. And this does not take into account manure, fertilizers, seed, pesticides and other expenses.

The Loss of Prestige of Traditional Food Crops

In traditional agrarian cultures, staple food crops have a prestige that reflects their central importance to the survival and well-being of the society. Similar to corn in the Andes of South America and rice in Asia, millet and sorghum were highly regarded by the people of the Sahelian countries. A number of religious practices and ceremonies revolved around planting and harvest tasks. They were the most used and valued commodities for trade, and nomads would exchange salt, leather, wool, spices and cowries[4] for grains. In the more humid forest regions of Ivory Coast, before coffee and cocoa became the major cash crops, rice and yam had the most prestige of the agricultural crops of most ethnic groups.

Among the Gourou, for example, rice was the most valued crop and food. Rice was cultivated by women, but was stored and placed under the control of the male head of the household [24]. It was used as a present and offered to guests and visitors. A wealthy man inevitably owned large quantities of rice. Yam was regarded as second to rice. Plantain had less prestige. Other vegetables were grown by women for sale, the proft being kept for their own use. Cassava, which originated from Latin America and was only recently established as a food crop, was considered as a food with low prestige because it could neither be stored nor transported easily. It was therefore unsuitable for accumulation or trade. It was also the property of women.

---

[4] Cowries were shells used as a currency in many parts of Africa for several centuries.

Table 1. A comparison of the prices of major staple foods in the Ivory Coast (1979–1985) [data from 30]

	Price/kg (francs CFA) mean for 1985	Price francs CFA/ 1,000 kcal	Relative price index/1,000 kcal	
			1979	1985
Imported rice	160	43.9	1.0	1.0
Manioc	73.7	67.7	1.61	1.54
Gari	184.3	94.0	1.62	2.14
Early yam	152.7	143.7	2.93	3.27
Late yam	104.4	80.9	2.12	1.84
Plantain	96.9	130.0	2.59	2.96

As economic reliance on cash crops increased, they became more central to the lives of the peasants. The low value placed on traditional grains by whites in the Sahel became reflected in the peasants' attitudes. This loss of prestige was accompanied by less production of millet and sorghum. It was also reflected in a lower consumption of millet and sorghum, especially in urban areas where they were considered less desirable than important foods [7]. Consequently, the contribution of traditional staple foods to the food supply of cities has deteriorated over the last decade. In Abidjan (Ivory Coast) in 1985, for example, the price of 1,000 kcal from local yam, cassava, 'gari', and plantain is one half to three times higher than 1,000 kcal from imported rice (table 1). The absence of protectionism for local farmers against the competition from imported wheat and rice has led to the stagnation of the traditional subsistence sector.

Cash Cropping in the Hands of West Africans

One of the reasons that prices of export crops from West Africa remained so low and actually declined since World War II is that almost all the production was in African hands. Although the colonial rule has not always been opposed to the attribution of concessions to expatriates, on many occasions, limitations were imposed to foreign firms or individual settlers. Moreover, almost all European plantations which were established in West Africa failed. According to Hopkins [15]:

They started with two serious drawbacks, a considerable ignorance of tropical conditions and a notable lack of capital. These handicaps often proved fatal at the outset. Even if they were overcome, two more problems arose almost immediately. The first was a shortage of labor, which also meant that wages had to be relatively high. The second problem was that plantations, being highly specialized, were particularly susceptible to shifts in world supply. Many of the early expatriate planters in West Africa committed themselves heavily to coffee production, and were eliminated by competition from South America soon after the turn of the century. Both problems are illustrated by the history of French plantations on the Ivory Coast, which survived in the form of forced labor and tariff preference. The record of expatriate plantations in the West African colonies was scarcely one to encourage either a very widespread demand for concessions, or wholehearted government support for European adventures in African agriculture.

The French government did not wish to faciliate the establishment of a large colony of settlers who were migrating in insufficient numbers to North Africa. West Africa was to be used as a source of raw materials for our industry and the inherent risks of agricultural production had to be borne by indigenous farmers. French or Lebanese traders were encouraged to purchase the available production but not often to invest in direct production. As Hopkins [15] shows, native peasant production had proved itself: Gold Coast, mostly from small producers, had become the first world exporters of cocoa by 1910. Senegambia, also from small native producers, had a well-established world market for its groundnut. The fact that the largest fraction of West Africa cash crop remained in African hands has had a considerable importance in the bargaining power of producers.

In dry tropical Africa, as Dumont [11] pointed out, the crops promoted during the colonial era, groundnut and cotton, provide only very low margins of profit. Almost never did any French colonizer cultivate either groundnut or cotton, leaving those crops to Africans, in order to dedicate his time to the more profitable business of trade or factory crop-processing. In the more humid Guinean forest region, coffee and cocoa cultivation offered opportunities for some accumulation of cash in the hand of Africans as early as the 1920s. In the Ivory Coast, a number of teachers, civil servants and even nurses and doctors rushed to take advantage of these new opportunities [35]. However:

In common with many areas of colonial Africa faced with worldwide depression in the 1930s, policies were instituted to discriminate against African smallholders. African cocoa was classified as 'wild' to permit collusion among purchasers to pay lower prices. Smallholders had difficulty in obtaining inputs, and bonus prices were allocated to holdof over 25 ha, thus excluding 99% of African producers. Furthermore, European planters were able to use forced labor ...

These conditions provided the barb for political organization among the southern Ivorian planters, united in opposition to forced labor despite the fact that they were personally exempt. The struggle ended in the suppression of forced labor in all French colonies in 1946 after a battle royal led in the French National Assembly by a young deputy who was to give his name to the law: Felix Houphouet-Boigny. Thus the history of cocoa in Ivory Coast is closely bound up with the creation of the Rassemblement Démocratique Africain, an offshoot of which is still the ruling party in Ivory Coast. Membership of the latter, at the highest levels, includes individuals with substantial cocoa interests. President Houphouet-Boigny, for example, maintains a cocoa farm of over 1,200 ha in Yamoussoukro ...

Despite the press attention attracted to the very large cocoa plantation in Ivory Coast, cocoa is overwhelmingly a smallholding product ... just under one person in five in Ivory Coast is directly involved in cocoa farming [35].

Recently, Gastellu and Affou Yapi [14] showed conclusively that a great number of people in the Ivorian power structure, including those in urban areas, have a direct financial stake in the health of the cocoa industry at the producer level. This is a significant difference between Ivory Coast and most other West African nations.

Relative Prices of Cash Crops and Food Crops in Two Sahel Countries

During the colonial era, prices paid to producers for their export crops were low. After the West African independence, prices of all export crops did not vary in the same way. Several indicators can be used to assess how the prices of cash crops have changed over time in relation to food prices, cost of living, wages, etc.

In Mali, over the postcolonial period of 1960–1983, the prices of the two major export crops, cotton and groundnut, have deteriorated in relation to that of millet or rice. The price for an equal weight of cotton was three times the price of millet in 1960–1961 and it fell to 1.4 in 1983. Groundnut prices were 1.4 times that of millet in 1960, it fell to 1 in 1982–1983 [21]. The priority given to cash crops in the 60s until the early 70s declined as the catastrophic food situation imposed a price increase of food crops.

In Burkina Faso [20], the change has been similar for cotton with a sharp decline of its price in relation to millet (from 2.75 to 1). Groundnut, which is predominantly a domestic food crop (less than 15% of national production is exported), has maintained its high price in relation to millet or even rice. The price ratio between domestic agricultural products and manufactured products affects the disparities in standard of living of agricultural versus nonagricultural population. Excessive disparities between rural and urban incomes may discourage farmers' activities.

In both Mali and Burkina Faso the disparity of income between peasants and urban dwellers is large. On the average nonagricultural incomes are six times higher than agricultural income. This is twice as large as in the majority of low-income countries and two and a half times what it is in Sri Lanka where a socialist government made efforts in favor of equity [19]. In addition, the concentration of investments and extension activities in the more fertile southern regions of Mali have increased regional disparities. From 1947 to 1959, out of a total investment of 14.4 million francs in agricultural development, the Office du Niger alone received 8.1 million (56%). All the resources designed to promote cash cropping in selected regions have created a class of farmers with intermediate income between urban and rural.

It was shown by Touya [39] that in the project area of the 'Compagnie Malienne pour le Développement des Textiles' (CMDT) in 1980-1981, the small farms had to give up cotton and grow maize instead: when the price of fertilizers increased faster than did that of cotton they could no longer take the risk. They could hardly produce enough grain for their own need and preferred to revert to food crops. Also, in the same study, Touya [39] indicated that the low price of cotton in Mali in recent years (1981) made this crop less profitable than millet or maize in relation to labor requirements: millet and sorghum pay twice as much per day's work as cotton, and maize four times as much as cotton.

Under these circumstances, it is understandable that the state agency had to offer a number of guarantees and services to maintain cotton cultivation. If prices of cotton and groundnut were deflated by prices of food crops only, the disadvantage of those cash crops would appear even more clearly because food prices have increased faster than the general price index. In view of this situation it seems that wherever peasants have the choice, their best interest is first to produce what they need for their own consumption, then to produce cereal for the market. If the present trends continue, grain cropping will continue to be more profitable than groundnut production at least. In Mali, both Operation Groundnut in 1967–1968 and Operation Groundnut and Food Crops (OACV) in 1973–1974 have failed. The failure of this last operation, backed by substantial resources, has increased the debt burden.

The New Patterns of Consumption

Colonialism and the ensuing dominant foreign presence brought with it cash cropping, monetarization and increased financial pressure on peasants and city dwellers. This led to the establishment of new patterns of consumption. Imported foods replaced traditionally sown staple grains. Sugar, vegetable oil, tomato paste, canned foods and alcoholic beverages became available everywhere. But agricultural commodities became a major expense on the national import bill. In 1964, Senegal spent 75 million US dollars, three quarters of the revenue from agriculture exports, to import rice and sugar, both of which could have been produced locally. Wheat alone, consumed by the urban minority, represented 6.6% of the import of agricultural products; wine, 2.3%; cheese, 0.9%; other milk products including butter, 5.1%; tea, 5.2%. Oranges were imported even though Senegal could produce a large variety of tropical fruits. Potato imports, consumed exclusively by the French and Senegalese bourgeoisie, accounted for 1.2%, or almost 1 million US dollars in 1964 [23].

In Dakar, in 1964, the equivalent in cash value of four fifths of the groundnut export were spent by the urban and provincial elite in eating a French-like diet. Bread from imported wheat, and flour, wine, cheese, milk and butter had a higher priority than water pumps, agricultural tools and other imports which could have raised the productivity of the traditional agricultural sector. Groundnut cultivation in itself was not the cause of social injustice, but only a means to extract from an arid and fragile environment resources which could then be concentrated in the hands of a small urban minority in Dakar and in France.

The case of wine import deserves special mention. 1.7 million US dollars worth of wine was imported to Senegal in 1964. Soon after the independence of French-speaking African states, Dumont [11] had already shown the danger of an increased wine and alcoholic beverage consumption in West Africa. The responsibility of French chambers of commerce as well as major wine dealers from Bordeaux and Marseille were denounced for many years. Until the mid-60s, wine was served in Dakar hospitals as part of the patient diet. Under the title, 'The Spread of Alcoholism', Dumont [11] wrote, in 1966:

After 1949, increases in wine and liquor imports took on frightening proportions. In 1951, fifteen times more liquor was imported to French West Africa than 1938, over three-quarters of a million gallons of pure alcohol. 1954 was a peak year for wine, the equivalent of 350,000 gallons of pure alcohol being imported. In 1953, 8% of the Ivory

Coast imports were alcoholic beverages. Wine and liquor monopolized up to 20% of the urban budgets of the Ivory Coast in 1954. The amount of money tied up in alcoholic beverages has never been estimated, but it is clearly enormous ... The flood of red wine pouring into the shanty towns is not an edifying sight either. Since the European is largely responsible for it, he has little to be proud of, particularly as he continues to set a bad example to African elites by having whiskey and champagne parties. The growth of African resources through FIDES[5] was in large measure sterilized by alcohol.

The labor of small farmers from Kaolack and Diourbel allowed the Senegalese and French bourgeoisie of Dakar to live in comfortable air-conditioned villas. While soils were gradually destroyed by not restoring the nutrients removed by monocropping, this bourgeoisie wasted precious revenue by building villas and offices, and in travels to Paris.

Nutritional Status of Senegalese Farmers

There is little information on the food situation of West African peasants before the period of independence. In general, the nutritional status of the Senegalese rural populations is better documented than that of the other Sahelian countries. The prevalent mediocrity of the nutritional status of the Senegalese population appears through various reports. In 1952, Bergouniou [4] found that, in the Dakar region, over 63% of the children examined showed some signs of nutritional deficiency, regardless of ethnic group. In a 1962 study, he found that prekwashiorkor was present in 4.6% of the children, reversible signs of malnutrition in 29% and other suggestive symptoms in 13% of the cases.

In 1962, Boutiller [5] found an average per capita intake of 2,200 kcal and 93 g of total protein, mostly from vegetable origin. ORANA[6] measured an intake of 2,200 kcal in January–April and 2,450 in August–November, which was estimated as slightly lower than the requirement. The diet was poor in protein, calcium, vitamin A, riboflavin, niacin and vitamin C (table 2). The French administration, with the assistance of a local staff, encouraged groundnut production in Senegal, which eventually absorbed half of the cultivated area. Meanwhile, in a 15-year period, the population grew by 59% and the production of basic foods per capita declined: from

[5] FIDES: 'Fond d'Investissement pour le Développement Economique et Social'.
[6] ORANA: 'Organisme pour la Recherche sur l'Alimentation et la Nutrition Africaines'.

Table 2. Nutrient intake of Senegalese Popenguine area, Senegal (1956) [data from 27]

Period	Calories	Anim. prot., g	Veg. prot., g	Fats g	Ca mg	Fe mg	Vit. A IU	Thiam. mg	Ribo. mg	Niac. mg	Vit. C mg
Jan.–April	2,200	11.1	48.77	32.5	515	17.1	457	1.90	0.44	4.5	42.4
	2,500	total prot. req. 87.67			1,180	12.4	4,515	1.17	1.85	11.8	77.9
	–12%	–32%			–56%		–90%		–76%	–61%	–45%
Aug.–Nov.	2,443	8.4	59.3	43.9	545	17.2	766	1.62	0.63	10.8	30.0
	2,461	total prot. req. 86.7			960	11.0	4,331	1.14	1.60	11.4	69.3
	–0.7%	–21.7%			–43%		–82%		–60%	–11%	–56%

Note: First line = findings by the investigators; second line = requirements computed on the basis of weight, sex, local conditions.
Deficiencies are computed as negative percentage of requirement. Adequate level intakes of other nutrients are not mentioned.

140 kg of millet and sorghum in 1948–1953 it dropped to 125 kg in 1964 and 121 kg in 1965 (–14%). If rice and corn are included with millet and sorghum, the per capita decline is from 170 kg in 1948 to 139 kg in 1965 (–6%). By contrast, the production of groundnut increased from 254 kg per capita (1945–1953) to 285 kg (+12%).

In the early 60s, a wide variety of nutritional diseases were reported in Senegal [23]. Numerous studies indicate the existence of widespread malnutrition and parasite infestation, especially in early childhood. Canterelle and N'Doye [23] observed mild forms of kwashiorkor and vitamin A deficiency in the Middle Valley of Senegal. Anemia was very common, as well as goiter; the average rate for the entire country was estimated at 3.6% but high prevalence could be found in areas such as Ziguinchore or Tambacounda. Payet et al. [29] observed beriberi in Basse Casamance and Pales [28] documented low levels of vitamin A in pregnant women. Bénéfice et al. [3] reported the results of several nutritional surveys conducted in Burkina Faso (1978), Southern Mali (1978, 1979), Northern Mali (1976) and Benin (1976). All villages investigated show some degree of infant malnutrition. Table 3 indicates the prevalence of moderate and severe forms of malnutrition in infants, children and adolescents, affecting more than 20%

Table 3. Prevalence of infantile and child malnutrition by age group and country in West Africa [data from 8]

Age group	Degree of malnutrition	Burkina Faso		Southern Mali		Northern Mali	Benin (Boukombe)	Senegal (Casamance)
		I	II	I	II			
0–1 year	n	57	184	45	51	83	47	40
	moderate	24%	20%	17%	20%	24%	8%	10%
	severe	3%	2%	2%	0%	1%	0%	0%
1–2 years	n	40	288	9	39	43	49	77
	moderate	37%	24%	11%	10%	30%	6%	5%
	severe	5%	1%	0%	0%	2%	0%	0%
2–6 years	n	223	433	68	159	62	31	220
	moderate	5%	11%	7%	4%	6%	0%	8%
	severe	1%	0%	1%	1%	0%	0%	0%

n = Number of children examined; moderate = 80 to 60% weight for height; severe = weight for height ≤ 60%.

Table 4. Percentage of adequacy of intake in reference to recommended allowances in six regions of Senegal [data from 8]

Region or city	Cal %	Prot. %	Ca %	Iron %	Vit. A %	Vit. B_1 %	Vit. B_2 %	Vit. PP %	Vit. C %
Dakar	96	154	42	83	81	77	39	176	223
Louga	95	158	52	121	54	92	44	186	249
Linguere	93	129	65	254	40	112	39	164	138
Diourbel	99	169	150	257	142	175	75	239	280
Casamance	98	137	70	191	387	105	42	190	223
Kedougou	78	114	89	174	87	140	48	192	240

of the children aged 15 and under. Chevassus-Agnès and Ndiaye [8] conducted five separate food consumption surveys in Senegal between 1977 and 1979. They conclude that in the diet of a large portion of the Senegalese population, energy intake per capita is low; calcium and riboflavin intakes are insufficient; retinol equivalents, folate and zinc are also present in insufficient amounts (table 4).

In conclusion, it appears that in Senegal, two distinct populations exist side by side, in terms of nutritional status and food intake: one of small farmers and rural dwellers who suffer from a wide spectrum of nutritional disorders and devote a large part of its work to groundnut production, and a second much smaller population living mostly in Dakar and Saint Louis, who consume imported rice, wheat, wine, cheese and dairy products. We have no published information on the nutritional status of this second privileged group. If nutritional disorders exist, it is improbable they are due to nutritional deficiencies.

Nutritional Status of Peasants from Burkina Faso

Contrary to the considerable expansion of groundnut in Senegal, in Burkina Faso (Upper Volta) cash cropping did not expand beyond 10% of the cultivated land. Therefore, its direct impact was probably less than that of the migration generated initially by forced labor and compulsory migration, and, later, by the need to earn money to meet social obligations by working in the Ivory Coast.

Burkina Faso is largely an eroded and overpopulated plateau with an average elevation of 800 feet above sea level. It was one of the most densely populated countries of West Africa and was therefore used as a reservoir of cheap labor for the other French West African colonies. At the time of independence in 1960, life expectancy was estimated to be only 32 years and literacy rates about 8%. This gives an indication of the level of priority health and education had during the colonial rule over Upper Volta[7]. For many years after colonization, cash cropping was not encouraged in Upper Volta for a number of reasons, including its excessive distance from the coast and shortage of available land. However, after World War II the cultivation of groundnut expanded from 167,000 hectares in 1948–1953 to 248,000 hectares in 1964–1965, at that time representing approximately 10% of the total land under cultivation at any one time of the year. Cotton did not reach 100,000 hectares until around 1950 and decreased thereafter. Almost all the cotton was exported, its price being so low that farmers had very little incentive to engage in cotton production.

---

[7] By contrast, according to Unesco, Kenya and Ghana had a much higher percentage of literate natives.

Table 5. Nutrients in the Kokoroue diets, Upper Volta (1953–1954) [data from 37]

Nutrients	Period			
	June–Oct.	Nov.–Feb. 15	Feb. 15–June 1	average
Calories consumed	2,424	1,680	2,448	2,147
Calories required	2,701	2,423	2,464	2,544
Percent of difference	– 10.3	– 3.7	– 0.7	– 15
Total proteins, g	78.4	46.6	74	65.3
Required	88	89	87	88
Percent of difference	– 11	– 48	– 15	– 30
Animal proteins, g	1.1	0.3	0.4	0.6

Note: The method used for the preparation of the table consisted of totaling the amount of foods consumed by all members of the study group during the entire study period regardless of age and sex. The requirements were based on the average temperature for the period considered and on the average weight of the participants. Other areas visited by the investigating team and inhabited by the same tribe included Ouahigouya, the Lake region, Doure, Tikare and Kossimoro. The results confirmed, in general, those found in Sinorosso. In two localities out of five (the Lake area and Tikare) the caloric intake was short (18 and 25.5%, respectively). The animal protein intake was very low in all five localities. Calcium intakes were short in all places [23].

In the early 50s, Serre [37] conducted a series of food consumption surveys on small samples of families from different ethnic groups. In all but one group he found that intake was below the recommended allowance (table 5). Among Gourmantche, in the District of Fada N'Gourma, total intake was 2,100 kcal, below the estimated requirement of 2,500 kcal. Total protein intake was adequate (72 g/day) but animal protein intake was very low (6,3 g/day). The diet of the Samogos families studied in the Tougan district was found to be low in calories (1,600 kcal instead of a recommended level of 2,600); total protein intake was 49 g and animal protein very low (0.82 g/day). Both in the Gourmantche and Somogo area, fat intake was low, respectively, 31 and 19 g/day. Consumption of the preferred foods, beans and groundnut, was very low: beans were present in only 6% of the meals, and groundnut, 1%.

Although these studies are not representative of the population at large, they add to the body of evidence that the average food intake of the rural population was grossly inadequate and there was a constant fear of

Table 6. Daily per capita energy intake in several regions of Mali (1971–1972) [data from 26, quoted in 21]

Region	Energy intake	Percent of energy requirement
South (cotton-growing region)	2,290	102
Center (groundnut-growing region)	1,780	79
West (groundnut-growing region)	1,500	67
MVNB (rice project region)	1,960	87
Delta (rice project region)	2,090	93
Office du Niger (rice and sugar cane)	2,310	103
Mean for above regions	1,990	88
Lakes and marshes (millet and cattle)	1,640	73
Upper valley (millet and sorghum)	1,800	80
Sahel (nomadic cattle)	1,770	79
Seno (millet and cattle)	2,100	93
Sixth region (cattle breeding)	1,420	63
Mean for above regions	1,750	78
Bamako (capital city)	2,610	116

food shortages of famine. In most countries of West Africa, the dietary intake of calories was low, the food was monotonous and poor in animal protein (table 2). This did not prevent the 'Institut de Recherche pour les Huiles et Oléagineux' (IRHO) and the 'Compagnie Française pour le Développement des Textiles' (CFDT) to extend the cultivation of groundnut and cotton for export on the best lands. However, the story of groundnut as a cash crop in Upper Volta has been that of a failure.

In Mali, a study conducted in 1971–1972 by Mondot-Bernard [26] provided some evidence of a higher food energy intake in cash cropping areas. Table 6 indicated that per capita energy intake was lower by 12% in noncash cropping areas, compared to the average intake in the six sets of villages from groundnut or cotton-growing regions. On the average, families studied in the cash cropping regions satisfied 88% of their estimated energy requirements. This was lower than in the capital city, Bamako, where per capita energy intake was 31% higher and estimated food energy requirements were met [21]. However, table 6 is misleading because regions where groundnut and cotton are cultivated are also those where rainfall is more abundant and reliable, and the infrastructure for cultivation and trade more developed. What is to be attributed to the earnings from cotton and groundnut cultivation and what is due to other economic, climatic or soil conditions is difficult to determine in the absence of further information.

Cash Cropping and Oil Revenue Increase Food Imports in Nigeria

In several West Africa countries (the Ivory Coast and Senegal, for example), the revenues from cash cropping have been used for massive imports of foreign foods. The neglect of traditional food crops, both by colonizers and the local bourgeoisie, associated with the new prestige, quality and convenient nature of imported food, has led to a decline of traditional food habits.

The same phenomenon did not occur in the groundnut production regions of Northern Nigeria, probably because they could import cereals from neighboring grain surplus areas and were somewhat protected by their distance from the sea. However, the flourishing revenues generated by the extraction of oil in the early 70s exaggerated the impact of cash cropping on food production. It caused a further decline of agricultural production and increased drastically food imports [2]. Between 1975 and 1983, two thirds of the foreign earnings expended on food imports by Nigeria were used for wheat and rice alone. Bread, which had become a staple food of the urban elite before 1975, became one of the most popular and cheapest foods. This, however, created a strong dependency on US grain suppliers. The drop in oil prices forced the Nigerian government to take steps to remedy the situation, by attempting to encourage local wheat production and by imposing a total ban on wheat imports as of January 1987. Despite a huge capital outlay, production of wheat from a large irrigation project has been a dismal failure [2].

Conclusion

The impact of cash cropping and export cropping on nutrition in West Africa cannot be examined out of its historical context. For three centuries, Dutch, Portuguese, Spanish, English and French slave traders shipped West Africans across the Atlantic because the cost of acquisition of slaves made it profitable to produce cash crops (sugar cane, tobacco, cotton and indigo) with imported labor in the Western Hemisphere (the Caribbean, Latin America and southeastern United States). It is estimated that 10–15 million men and women and children were uprooted from their native land for the production of goods sought by European industrialists. As captives, West Africans received the bare minimum to survive the transatlantic trip, reproduce and work. The high demand for tropical products in Europe generated in Africa a considerable amount of human suffering, social disorganization and the gradual destruction of several major West African kingdoms.

For many years after West Africa was brought under military domination, local chiefs had to supply 'forced labor' to construct roads, railways, storehouses and administrative buildings meant to transport, house or organize the production of cash crops. Cash cropping existed on a small scale before colonization and even before trade developed with Europe. However, monocropping, as it became prevalent in Senegal and Gambia, or reliance on a few cash crops, as it occurred in the Ivory Coast, Ghana, Mali or Equatorial Guinea, was the direct result of colonial domination and influence.

It is a rather jesuit argument to separate, as some supporters of cash cropping do, the impact of colonial rule from that of cash cropping per se. One was the justification for the other. Nor is it necessary to be a believer of the myths of a 'merry Africa' in precolonial time to imagine that Africa's destiny could have been better without slavery and colonization. Citing these obvious facts is often coined polemical in academic circles.

West Africans, until the era of African independences, were unable to negotiate the price paid for their work or their products. Inasmuch as small producers remained largely scattered over large territories, were isolated, uneducated and not organized into cooperatives or unions, the traders maximized their profits by paying the lowest possible price for export crops. In order to maintain cash crop prices at the lowest possible level, all other prices affecting the cost of living also had to be kept low. Since wage labor was required for either planting, harvesting, transporting and processing cash crops, staple food had to be made available at a cheap cost.

This rationale led to sizable imports of rice from Indochina to Senegal but also to a number of measures to improve cereal production, storage and trade in the Sahel countries. As men migrated, staple food prices were kept low by maintaining the responsibility for their food supply in their native villages. For example, in Upper Volta, the women remained in the villages while the adult men were employed in the Ivory Coast or in major cities. Their unpaid work was used to produce the millet and sorghum to feed the laborers (thus preventing what would otherwise be the responsibility of plantation owners to provide food). In addition, the modern sector (cities and plantations) obtained from the subsistence sector laborers for which it had not paid any social expense and in most cases would not pay any pension. Since colonial times, the subsistence sector has subsidized the modern market sectors by supplying the productive workers at zero cost. Before and after their productive age, those workers, as children and then as old invalid workers, were fed by their villages of origin [6].

Cash cropping in West Africa remained predominantly in the hands of Africans. A number of plantations by Europeans failed and large production schemes by private or public investors proved too costly to be profitable. The fact that few Europeans invested in tropical production and when they did they selected different crops and different production techniques than Africans, resulted in large part from two factors. First, the prices paid to Africans for their cash crops were low and very few Europeans would have lived on it. Second, the major margins of profit were made in the processing and trade, not in the production. This division of labor allowed Europeans to underpay producers for many decades. The low income of most African producers had two major negative outcomes: the great difficulty for them to save and invest enough in order to raise productivity, and a low standard of living which included poor health and nutrition.

Their isolation, their lack of Western type of education, the financial pressure exerted by the economic and administrative environment has led to a poorly productive use of the earnings form cash cropping. Added to the rising individual taxes to be paid to the government, the numerous obligations of peasants, the weddings and other celebrations and solidarity of the extended family soon swallowed the earnings from cash cropping. Not only were savings and productive investments not encouraged and taught to peasants, but in addition a Western pattern of consumption was imposed in all possible ways (advertising, credit, example of the elites, etc.). The dominant consumption model placed on a pedestal included bread, rice, condensed milk, beer, wine, brandy and whisky, canned food and a number of other foods which gradually displaced traditional food crops [12]. Cash cropping became gradually one of the few means to acquire preferred goods, such as radios, watches, bicycles, and clothes. The revenues from cotton, groundnut, coffee, cocoa, palm oil, etc. have spent very little time in the hands of cash crop growers.

The same trading companies that flourished in Liverpool, Amsterdam, Nantes and Bordeaux from slave trade in the 18th century, gave birth to major trading companies who invested in the legitimate trade with West Africa in the middle of the 19th century.

The trade of vegetable oil between West Africa and Europe led to the expansion of Unilever, which in turn invested in export of manufactured goods to West Africa. A close alliance often existed between banks which invested in West Africa, major trading companies, and dominant lobbies represented in the Parliament in Paris. Governors in Abidjan and Dakar were ordered to undertake civil works which directly benefited French investors. Forced labor was placed at the disposal of agricultural enterprises, and district commissioners had a privileged relationship with French traders from whom they would get all their supplies and a number of services. Lebanese shopkeepers acting as intermediaries created a network of grocery shops, drugstores and fabric, clothes and shoe shops which offered in the most remote sectors all the manufactured goods France could export to West Africa. Specific efforts were made at the time of the harvest to capture the largest fraction of the domestic earnings from cash crop sales. Alcoholic beverages managed to drain a sizable portion of urban and rural income, even in some Moslem-dominant regions.

All this appears today inevitable and very few of us imagine that it could have been any different. To compare, as some researchers have done, the food situation of cash croppers with noncash croppers in a context where only cash croppers are assisted is a biased and unfair comparison. For more than a century now, subsistence growers have been at a disadvantage compared to export or cash croppers.

The availability of land, population density and rainfall in the Sahelian, the Sudanian and the Guinean regions of West Africa dictated very different solutions to the combined cultivation of food crops and cash crops. Among the Baoule tribe in the Ivory Coast, the forest would be cleared to cultivate cassava and tobacco, and then used for coffee the following years. There was no conflict in the seasonal demand for work and it remained possible for farmers to grow both food crops and cash crops jointly or in sequence. However, the intense erosion resulting from this system threatened to reduce the productivity of a large extension of arable land. Coffee and cocoa cultivation led to excessive deforestation, soil degradation and forced farmers to migrate to new regions and open new colonization areas. On the other hand, the lack of technological advances on traditional food crops (cassava, yam, plantain and to some extent corn and beans) made the cultivation of those crops unprofitable.

Until recent years, a very limited effort had been made in favor of African food crops. The short storage life and long processing of cassava and yams has constituted severe limiting factors to the extension of these crops. Presently, they are at a great disadvantage compared to wheat and rice. The limited improvement of most varieties of Afrian staple foods and the lack of a prestigious food industry based on these products naturally lead to the adoption of industrial products from Western industry based on wheat, potato, corn or rice products. Cash cropping in the humid part of Africa has not discouraged the production of traditional food crops, but it has made it less prestigious. In addition, it has seldom been a profitable business and few Europeans have invested in staple food production in the Ivory Coast, Benin or Togo.

In Sahelo-Sudanian regions, groundnut and cotton on one side and millet and sorghum on the other have been in direct competition in many instances: good, arable land is limited; colonizers imposed cultivation on the best lands. Since there is only one rainy season in the Sahelian countries, peasants had to decide what to cultivate first. Early sowing would increase significantly the likelihood of a good harvest. Too early sowing would increase the risk of insufficient rains and might force peasants to sow again. In any event, cash cropping competed for land and labor with food crops. The decline of per capita millet and sorghum production while groundnut production increased in Senegal (1950–1975) and the record production of cotton of the Sahel countries (1983–1984) while food imports reached a peak [38] are not mere coincidences.

The World Bank quotes, whenever necessary, the concomitant increase of food crops and cash crops in a number of African countries but this is not the case in the Sahel countries. Moreover, the increase in per capita food production of some countries does not exclude the fact that cash crops have been grossly underpaid, nor that the profitable part of crop processing had been kept in the hands of Western multinationals. In addition, the pressure from the IMF and the World Bank to increase production of most cash crops is highly questionable in view of the projected deterioration of world prices of most tropical export crops in the coming decade.

Forecasts for prices elaborated by the World Bank for a number of agricultural products for 1995 are not optimistic. They should rise considerable concern among coffee, cotton, rice, rubber and sorghum export countries, and a number of others. Agricultural export-driven development has led many tropical countries to a deadlock. What Africa needs is profound economic reorientation geared at the creation of a West African market. It would be based on regional complementarity, protectionism for young local industries and aim at the satisfaction of basic needs.

In that respect, African leaders should study meticulously how the Chinese central and provincial governments had in the 1960s: (a) given priority to regional self-sufficiency in grain; (b) limited the cultivation of preferred food and cash cropping in order to ensure an adequate staple food supply; (c) educated as rapidly and as effectively as possible the rural masses; (d) raised producer prices of staple foods at the expense of urban consumers in order to stimulate production; (e) prevented the sale of any luxury goods but on the contrary made all basic goods and services available to the masses, and (f) adopted many other measures which have reduced drastically rural poverty and malnutrition and limited rural-urban income disparities.

When one considers that nothing approaching those steps has ever had a high degree of priority in any of West African colonized territorries, one feels that West Africa has adopted policies which are often inappropriate to ensure an adequate food supply in the future.

Cash cropping is closely linked to the persistence of a dependent model of development. Malnutrition is only one manifestation of the unfair distribution of income and the inappropriate use of public and private earnings provided by agricultural domestic trade and exports.

Contemporary economists who analyze the impact of cash cropping and export cropping in Africa often fail to recall the logic and historical context of the expansion of the modes of production they implied. Asking nowadays, 'under what conditions is the expansion of export cropping a favorable impact on nutrition?' is not a question which is as open-ended as it sounds. The answer must start by the clear recognition that our trade links with most African states are based on their export crops. Their roads and railway networks, their agricultural research stations, their banking systems have been raised over export and cash cropping. For a farmer to decide to produce livestock or food crop for local industries instead of export crops is like swimming upstream in a context which is organized primarily for export cropping.

Cash cropping had detrimental effects which are more apparent under two circumstances. The first is when the extension of cash cropping has been done at the expense of traditional staple grains which were already in short supply. Such has been the case in southern Niger (Maradi). The second is when farmers were not organized nor connected to a responsible extension agency; such was the case of groundnuts in Upper Volta (Burkina Faso). In contrast, cash cropping in the Guinean zone often did not compete with staple root or tuber crops. In the Ivory Coast, cocoa growers were both able to control a large segment of the ruling party and to directly benefit from the trade of their main cash crops when world prices were favorable (table 7).

Table 7. Examples of differences in the income and food impact of cash cropping in West Africa

Ecological region	Sahelo-Sudanian		Guinean	
Rainfall	scanty, irregular		abundant, sufficient quantity	
Vegetation	savanna and wooded steppe		tropical rain forest and woodland	
Food crops	millet, sorghum, corn		rice, cassava, yam, plantain	
Cash crops	cotton, groundnut		coffee, cocoa, plam oil	
Example selected	Mali	Burkina Faso	Ivory Coast	Ghana
Cash crop selected	cotton	groundnut	cocoa	cocoa
Growers' association	organized farmers by CMDT	absence of grower's association	farmer's lobby influential in National ruling party	weakness of farmer's association
Cash crop expansion	only small farms are unable to cultivate both cotton and food grains; cotton increases yields	as in South Niger groundnut expansion is in conflict with sorghum and millet; groundnut lowers yields	cocoa does not conflict with staple food	cocoa has limited conflict with basic food staples
Income	increased income	stagnation of income	marked increase in income	reduction in cocoa production
Food intake and nutrition	improved food intake and nutrition	groundnut revert to food crop-stagnation of food intake	improved food intake	stagnation of food intake

A small number of studies have shown that in regions where both cash cropping and traditonal food cropping are practiced, cash croppers frequently have a higher income and sometimes a better nutritional status. The conclusions which can be derived from such comparisons should always be placed in the correct perspective. In an economic system which is organized around cash cropping as a mechanism for surplus extraction, it is logical that cash croppers should be, at least on the average, slightly better off than noncash croppers. This, in turn, is not in contradiction with the essence of the system. The real issue is not whether in such a system, farmers should or should not practice cash cropping: they often have little choice. Unless we envision the possibility of altering the nature of the relationship of farmers to the state apparatus, there is very little leeway for action. Both de Janvry [16] and Mellor [25] have stressed the role of powerful producer associations in the improvement of the conditions of cash croppers. The increase in income of cocoa growers in the Ivory Coast or cotton growers in southern Mali is due to the links of these farmers to the ruling party. de Janvry [16] points out that a strong political representation of farmers is a fundamental prerequisite of the improvement of their condition:

> The safeguard of those interests requires more than the social integration by which farmers have access to credit, information, markets, and so forth. It requires their political integration, enabling farmers to become full-fledged citizens in the political apparatus and to assert their rights through lobbying groups.

One can predict that the increased participation of farmers' associations to the decision process at the central level of planning would lead to major alterations in the investment priorities and the allocation of resources.

The formulation of new strategies will inevitably reflect the balance of power between the various actors of the political apparatus. Once the farmers have established their control over part of the national budget, they will obtain a better allocation of resources between production for the domestic market and for export. They need central or cooperative institutions to buffer the adverse effects of drought or rapid changes of prices on the world market. They need appropriate price policies to stimulate domestic production, etc. Gradually the nature of the present cash cropping system will be modified and farmers will capture the urban food market. Presently, the urban market is largely supplied by imports and benefits little the local producers. A shift towards increased self-sufficiency with appropriate price policies can give local peasants a broader and more advantageous set of options.

Summary

The impact of cash cropping in West Africa cannot be isolated from its social and historical background. Among the many changes brought to West African economies by cash cropping since the beginning of the century, the present document shows how the extension of trade with European merchants and colonizers created new sets of values and criteria for wealth. Food crops gradually lost their prominent cultural and economic roles to the benefit of export crops or goods.

Traditional systems of agricultural production were profoundly disrupted by military actions. They imposed colonial rule and control of trade of tropical crops and goods.

Forced labor and compulsory (poorly paid) work assignments were instituted for private and public enterprises: construction of roads, railways, public buildings and plantations. The main justification was the need for cheap labor to cultivate, transport and build roads for the extraction of raw materials. This in turn caused massive migrations from countries such as Burkina Faso (Upper Volta) to Ivory Coast.

Cash cropping made systematic collection of taxes possible. An imposition on a per capita basis became the rule and the major incentive of small farmers to engage in commercial farming. Cash cropping made also possible extensive monetarization of West Africa. This results in both favorable and unfavorable effects on the quality of the diet. In profoundly disrupted traditional societies, the diffusion of new consumption patterns was easier and faster. It led to massive food imports of wheat, rice, sugar, alcohol, etc. Cash cropping was (and still is) practiced as a 'mining' agriculture, exhausting soils and deteriorating their fertility for extended periods of time.

In the Sudanian and Sahelian zones cash cropping conflicted with the cultivation of grains because peak demands for labor were similar. Therefore, millet and sorghum production declined. Cash cropping was developed in response to the need of European economies for tropical products. However, colonization as a tool to obtain these raw materials was highly inefficient and associated with a considerable misuse of public funds. Together with cash cropping extension was created a network of intermediaries of large European corporations and shopkeepers who would efficiently drain all the earnings from cash cropping away from productive agricultural investments. It made possible the birth of local bourgeoisies and states dedicated almost exclusively to the extraction of a surplus value from the peasantry through cash cropping. It led to a displacement of the role of women; by attributing to them the less profitable food crops, the new production system managed to feed local cities and migrant workers at low cost. Cash cropping provides indirectly a new mean of exploiting women's labor.

Cash cropping by small independent producers is also associated with a stagnation of labor productivity. Mostly because the production and trade systems do not favor capital accumulation at the domestic producer's level. Concentration of the risk of crop failure and price deterioration remained at the peasant's level. Foreign firms invest almost no capital and local elites often prefer to send the profits of their sales of cash crop to a foreign bank account, rather than to invest it in domestic agriculture. Following the example of colonizers, a large majority of local bourgeoisies and West African states have used cash cropping to squeeze from agriculture a maximum flow of resources. In doing so they have often jeopardized the growth of that sector and the rest of the economy. The stagnation of agriculture has, in turn, drastically reduced its capacity to adequately feed a growing population.

References

1   Afana, O.: L'économie de l'Ouest africain: perspective de développement (Maspero, Paris 1966).
2   Andrae, G.; Beckman, B.: The wheat trap. Bread and underdevelopment in Nigeria. Zed Book, London, UK, in Association with the Scandinavian Institute of African Studies, Uppsala, Sweden, 1985, reported in Food Policy, p. 284 (Aug. 1987).
3   Bénéfice, E.; Chevassus-Agnès, S.; Barral, H.: Nutritional situation and seasonal variations from a pastoralist population of the Sahel (Senegalese Ferlo). Ecol. Food Nutr. *14:* 229–247 (1981).
4   Bergouniou, J.: Malnutrition et sous-nutrition chez les jeunes enfants de la presqu'île du Cap-Vert (en dehors) de Dakar. Bull. Méd. AOF Fr. *9:* 1 (1952).
5   Boutiller, J.L., et al.: La moyenne vallée du Sénégal (Ministère de la Coopération, Paris 1962).
6   Brun, T.A.; Bleiberg, F.: Cereal shortages and adjustment in the Sahel. Food Policy *5:* 3 (1980).
7   Brun, T.; Dupin, H.: Les paysans du Tiers-Monde ne fabriquent plus leur nourriture et achètent du Coca-Cola. Croissance des Jeunes Nations (Paris, 1974).
8   Chevassus-Agnès, S.; Ndiaye, A.M.: Enquête de consommation alimentaire de l'ORANA de 1977 à 1979: méthodes et résultats; in Etat nutritionnel de la population du Sahel. Rapport d'un groupe de travail, France, 1980, (IDRC-160F, Ottawa 1981).
9   Dewey, K.G.: Agricultural development, diet and nutrition. Ecol. Food Nutr. *8:* 265 (1979).
10 Dewey, K.G.: Nutritional consequences of the transformation from subsistence to commercial agriculture in Tabasco, Mexico. Human Ecol. *9:* 151–187 (1981).
11 Dumont, R.: False start in Africa (Praeger, New York 1966).
12 Dupin, H.; Brun, T.: Evolution de l'alimentation dans les pays en voie de développement. Cah. Nutr. Diét. *8:* 4 (1973).
13 Fleuret, P.; Fleuret, A.: Nutrition, consumption and agricultural change. World Bank, Working Paper Series, 65 (1980).
14 Gastellu, J.M.; Affou Yapi, S.: Un mythe à décomposer: la bourgeoisie de planteurs, pp. 149–180; in Faure Y.A., Médard, J.-F. (eds): Etat et bourgeoisie en Côte d'Ivoire (Karthala, Paris 1981).
15 Hopkins, A.G.: An economic history of West Africa (Columbia University Press, New York 1973).

16   Janvry, A. de: Dilemmas and options in the formulation of agricultural policies in
     Africa; in Gettinger, J., Leslie, J., Hoisington, C. (eds): Food Policy. EDI Series
     (John Hopkins University Press, New York 1987).
17   Kayser, B.: L'agriculture et la sociéte rurale des régions tropicales (SEDES, Paris
     1969).
18   Kennedy, E.: Effect of cash crop production on household production, consump-
     tion and decision-making: some theoretical considerations (IFPRI, Washington
     1986).
19   Lecaillon, J.; Morrison, C.; Schneider, H.; Thorbeke, E.: Politiques économiques et
     performances agricoles dans les pays à faible revenu (OCDE, Paris 1987).
20   Lecaillon, J.; Morrisson, C.: Politiques économiques et performances agricoles: le
     cas du Burkina Faso, 1960–1983 (OCDE, Paris 1986).
21   Lecaillon, J.; Morrisson, C.: Politiques économiques et performances agricoles: le
     cas du Mali, 1960–1983 (OCDE, Paris 1986).
22   Lev, L.: The effect of cash cropping on food consumption adequacy among the Meru
     of Northern Tanzania. Working Paper No. 21 (Michigan State University, East
     Lansing 1981).
23   May, J.M.: The ecology of malnutrition in West Africa, and Madagascar (Hafner,
     New York 1968).
24   Meillassoux, C.: Anthropologie économique des Gourous de Côte-d'Ivoire (Mouton,
     Paris 1964).
25   Mellor, J.W.: A structural view of policy issues in African agricultural development
     (IFPRI, Washington 1984).
26   Mondot-Bernard, J.: Analyse de la situation alimentaire en Afrique. Rapport final,
     Plan quinquenal, Mali (Centre de Développement OCDE, Paris 1974).
27   ORANA: Organisme de Recherche sur l'Alimentation et la Nutrition africaine.
     Enquête Alimentaire de Popenguine (Dakar, 1956).
28   Pales, L.: Alimentation et nutrition. Rapports No. 1–3 (Direction Générale de la
     Santé Publique, Dakar 1947).
29   Payet, M.; et al.: Société médicale d'Afrique noire de Langue française. Presse méd.
     68 (1969).
30   Perrault, P.; Tano, K.: Commercialisation des vivriers à Abidjan. Rapport final
     (CIRES, Abidjan 1986).
31   Pinstrup-Andersen, P.: The impact of export crop production on human nutrition;
     in Biswas, M., Pinstrup-Andersen, P. (eds): Nutrition and Development (Oxford
     University Press, Oxford 1985).
32   Raynaut, C.: Le cas de la région de Maradi (Niger); in Copans (ed): Sécheresse et
     famines au Sahel. Dossiers Africains (Maspero, Paris 1975).
33   Rodney, W.: How Europe underdeveloped Africa (Tanzania Publishing House, Dar-
     es-Salaam 1972).
34   Sarraut, A.: La mise en valeur des colonies françaises (Paris 1923); see also Sarraut,
     A.: La mise en valeur des colonies françaises (Paris 1949) in ref. [36].
35   Sawadogo, P.: Impact de la croissance démographique sur le développement écono-
     mique et social en République de Côte-d'Ivoire. Population et économie de Côte-
     d'Ivoire (Nations Unies; Commission Economique des Nations Unies pour l'Afri-
     que, Abidjan I 1980).

36 Schreyer, E.: L'Office du Niger au Mali. La problématique d'une grande entreprise agricole dans la zone du Sahel (Steiner, München 1983).

37 Serre, A.: Enquête alimentaire en Haute-Volta, vol. 1–5 (ORANA, Dakar 1952).

38 Timberlake, L.: Africa in crisis: the cause, the cure of environmental bankrupcy. (International Institute for Environment and Development, London 1985).

39 Touya, J.C.: Influence de la politique des prix sur les performances agricoles de la région de Koutiala (Mali) zone CMDT; in Lecaillon, J., Morrisson, C. (eds): Politiques économiques et performances agricoles: le cas du Mali, 1960–1983 (OCDE, Paris 1986).

T.A. Brun, PhD, Institut Agronomique Méditerranéen
Route de Mende, F–34000 Montpellier (France)

Subject Index

Colonization effects on cash cropping
127–159
Coronary heart disease
alcohol consumption effects
blood pressure 47, 48, 52–54
case-control studies 42–44
cholesterol metabolism 48–50,
54–56
cohort studies 44–47
dependence of drinking level 44–47
haemostasis 50, 51, 56–60
occlusion score when correlated to
smoking 43, 44
ten-year mortality rates 45
inverse relationship to alcohol
consumption in ecological studies
39–41
mortality rate 39, 45
risk factors 39, 47, 48, 50
Creatine phosphokinase, activity increase
after extreme work load 94
Creatinine, level after extreme work load
92, 94

Dental caries
adult population trend 2
cariogenic potential models 5, 6, 10
effect of salivation level 24, 25
effects of delivery media of sweeteners
10, 22, 23
fluoride effect 2, 23
importance of consumption frequency
in animal studies 21
natural defense mechanisms 23
rat similarity to humans 15, 21
role of sugar in development 1, 2
sorbitol cariogenicity 10, 11
see also Sorbitol
Dietary intake, factors in athletes 72, 73
see also Extreme work load

Extreme work load
citrate synthetase activity increase 82,
83
creatine phosphokinase activity
increase 94
danger of high protein intake 95

energy output during 81, 92
factors effected before, during and after
exercise
apolipoprotein level 81, 83
blood lactate level 81, 82
calcium intake 78, 86, 92
carbohydrate intake 77, 87, 91, 93,
94
cholesterol level 81, 83, 88, 89
creatinine level 92, 94
energy intake 76, 85, 90
fat intake 77, 80, 81, 87, 91, 93, 94
glycemia level 81, 82
hematocrit level 83, 84
high density lipoprotein level 81, 83,
88, 89
iron intake 78, 86, 92
low density lipoprotein level 81, 83,
88, 89
nonesterified fatty acid level 88, 89
oxygen consumption 74, 75
PP factor intake 80, 86, 92
protein intake 76, 77, 87, 89, 91, 93,
94
triglyceride level 81, 83, 92
urea level 82, 83, 88, 89, 92, 94, 95
uric acid level 82, 83, 88, 89, 94, 95
vitamin
A intake 79, 86, 92
B_1 intake 79, 86, 92
B_2 intake 79, 86, 92
C intake 80, 86, 92
hydroxyacetyl-CoA-dehydrogenase
activity increase 82, 83
mean running velocity in twenty-four
hour run 74, 75
normal parameters after recovery 84,
96
nutritional parameters from
climbing 91–94
intensive training 94, 95
triathlon 84–91
twenty-four hour run 74–84
participant
body mass index 74, 85, 90
lean body mass 74, 85, 90
trend in sports competition 73